MW00812241

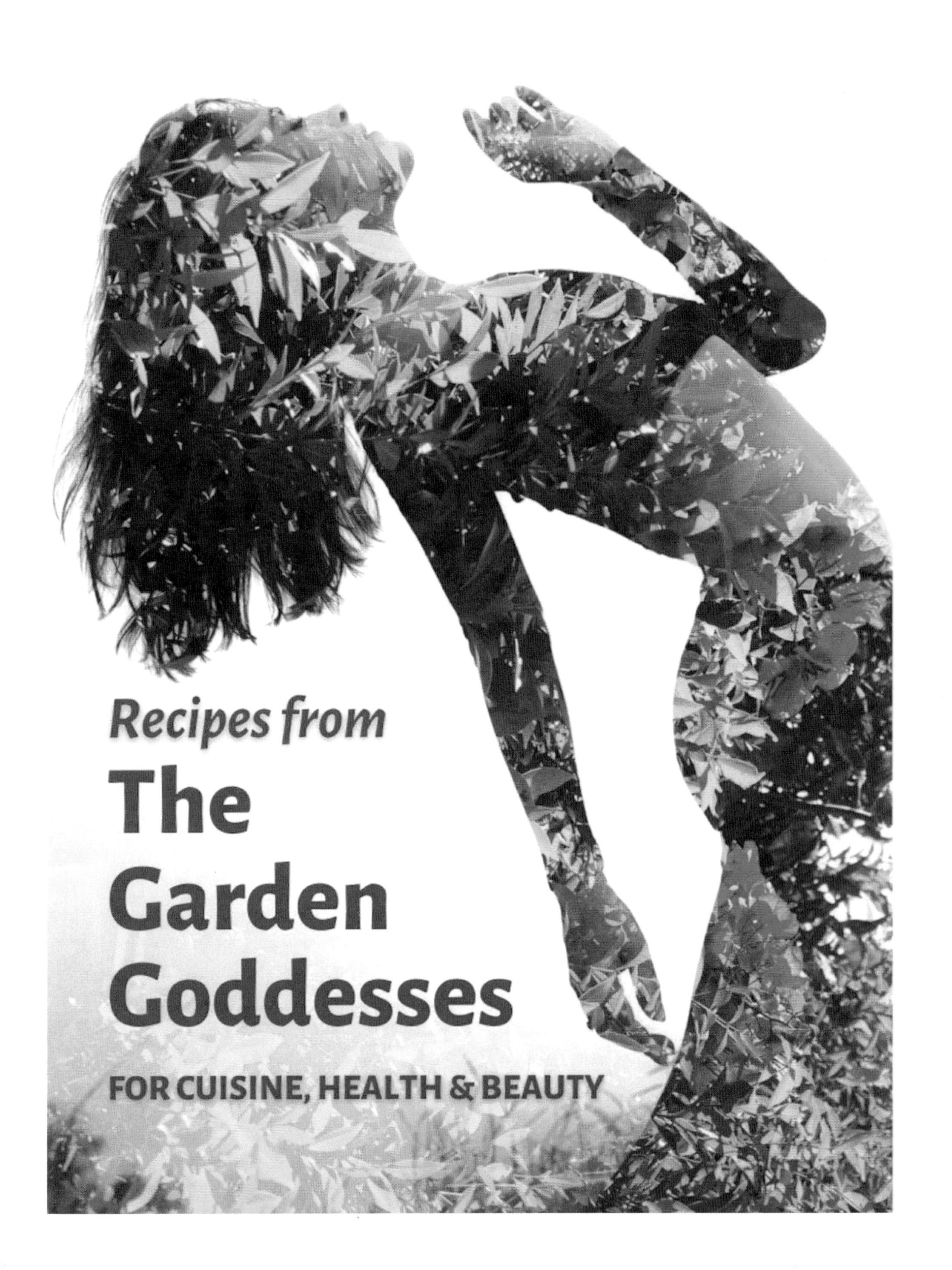

Recipes from

The Garden Goddesses

FOR CUISINE, HEALTH & BEAUTY

The information in this book is intended for educational/entertainment purposes only and recipes should not be considered as a recommendation or an endorsement of any particular medical or health treatment. Please consult a health care provider before pursuing any herbal treatments or recipes shared in this book. You are responsible for your own health.

Published by: The Society of Garden Goddesses® in collaboration with From Pen to Published
Photographer: Dana Stevens
Book & Cover Design: Mariah Miller Creative Services

First edition: 2023
Paperback ISBN: 979-8-9890003-0-2

Acknowledgments: All photos copyrighted and taken by Susan Gouveia and Dana Stevens Photography, except:
pg. i: used with permission of author; ii: @Rimma_Bondarenko, Getty Images
pg. 24: @olga miltsova/karandev, Getty Images; 25: @romiri, Getty Images; 26: @lauriepatterson, Getty Images
pg. 32: @adamcalaitzis, Getty Images; 33: @olgamitsova, Getty Images; 35 @gajus
pg. 37: center photo @monikagrabkowska, unsplash
pg. 39-41: ©Heather Brassfield
pg. 50: @ildipapp; 51: @pixelshot, @jon11, Getty Images; 52: @olgachzhu, @yuliyafurman, @nata_vkadsidey; @illiyaka minetsky; 53: @altastudio, @vm2002; 54: @leostein, Getty Images; 55: @grafvision, Getty Images
pg. 61: ©Gina Vian; 63: @homydesign; 64: @trirbickis, Getty Images; 65: ©Gina Vian; 66: @solphoto, Getty Images; 67: @vm2002
pg. 75: ©Mila Johansen; 74: ©Dana Stevens; 75: anamomarques, Getty Images; 77-82: Deposit Photos; 83: ©Mila Johansen, top right: @leonori, Getty Images, bottom right: @dariayakovieva, Pixabay
pg: 88: ©Miriam Lytle; 89: @dny59, Getty Images; 90: @msphotographic, Getty Images; 91: @bhofack2, Getty Images; 92: @styxclick, Getty Images; 93: ©Miriam Lytle
pg. 95: @choonsmin63, Getty Images; 96: restock images
pg. 101: @lesliebrienza, Getty Images; 102: @mariha-kitchen, Getty Images; 103: @vaphotog, Getty Images
pg. 106: ©Donna Abreu; 108: @lum3n, Pexels; 110: Dreamstime; freestock.org, Pexels; 111: @bhofad2, Getty Images; 113: @elenaphoto; 116: ©Donna Abreu; 117: @gabrannon, getty images; 118: ©Donna Abreu;
pg. 121: @tomhendricks, Getty Images; @carlosrojas20, Getty Images
pg. 128-135: ©Dana Stevens Photography, 136: ©Gale Pylman; wings: @richarddavies, apex creations; flower: @sparklestroke; 141: @kerdkanko, Getty Images
pg. 153: @madeleinesteinbach; 154: Elizabeth McLeod; 155: @pixelshot; 156: @artstudioimages; 157: E. McLeod;
pg. 159, 162, 163: ©Brian Johnson; 164-171: ©Elizabeth Flores Pantoja
pg. 174: Artist: Masha Lewis, ©The Society of Garden Goddesses®
Author bio photos by Dana Stevens Photography and are copyrighted.

This book is dedicated with deep gratitude
to all of the Garden Goddesses
who have contributed their knowledge, creativity, and
fabulous potluck dishes to our 500+ gatherings since 2010.
May we all continue to inspire you in your creative, healthy,
and happy gardens, kitchens, and community!

Table of Contents

FOREWORD

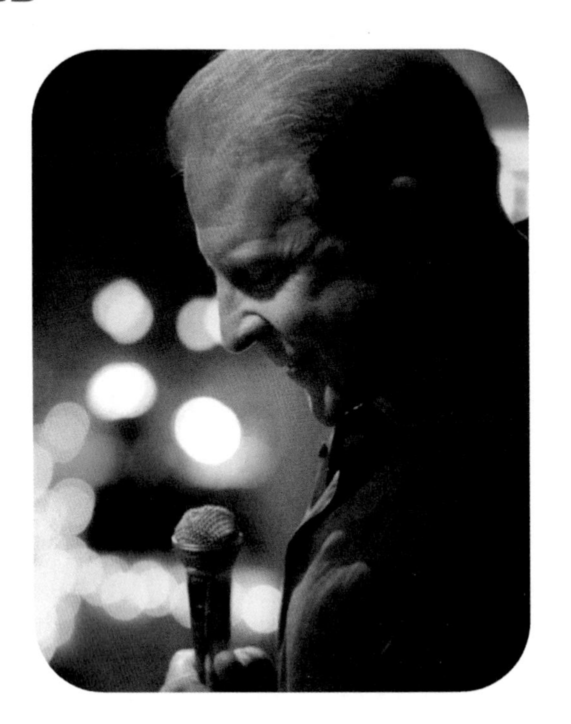

One of the nicest things you can feel about a person is that they are "down to earth."

Which, in turn, says a lot about the colossal value of earth.

When it came time in history to feed humans, the earth offered up its bountiful gifts to give us creatures everything we needed.

Vitamins and minerals and nutrients.

Food is medicine.
Food is fun.
Food is delicious.
Did I say fun?

We can retrain our taste buds.
To not crave toxic food.
To enjoy the delectable and immense flavors of real food from the earth.
That dance in the light of the moon.

Food becomes more luscious when prepared with love.
It sounds corny and it is.
And true.

This book of recipes is a compilation of love and beauty and fun.
Made by a group of passionate and compassionate humans who marinate in the beauty of the earth.
People who respect themselves and the planet.
Who ensure their family and friends are well cared for.

The salt of the earth!

Eddie Brill
Comedian, actor, writer, producer and plant lover!

Eddie Brill's Creamsicle Smoothie

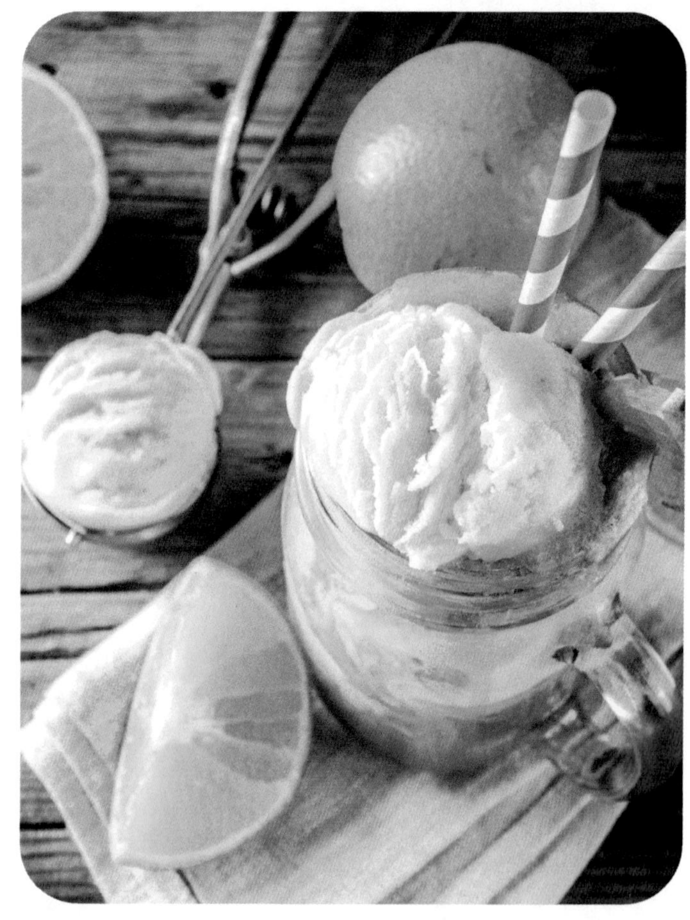

Our family has always been in love
with ice cream.
And now that we have sampled
vegan ice-cream, we are
Going to marry ice cream.

Not the processed in your grocer's
freezer vegan ice cream,
but freshly made with nature's
heavenly ingredients.
We love vegan ice cream that is
coconut based.
Although I once had hemp-based
vegan chocolate ice cream
and mmm mmm mmm, my dish
ran away with the spoon.

We grew up with very little money yet bursting with love. Our biggest treat was our once-a-week trip to the local ice cream parlor. Yet, occasionally we would make our own concoctions at home.

One of our family's favorite, yet simplest recipes basically creates a creamsicle.

Mix vegan vanilla bean ice cream with fresh-squeezed oranges and a small handful of ice in a blender. Do not blend for more than 45 seconds.

Add love!

INTRODUCTION

Meet Susan Gouveia

By Valerie Costa

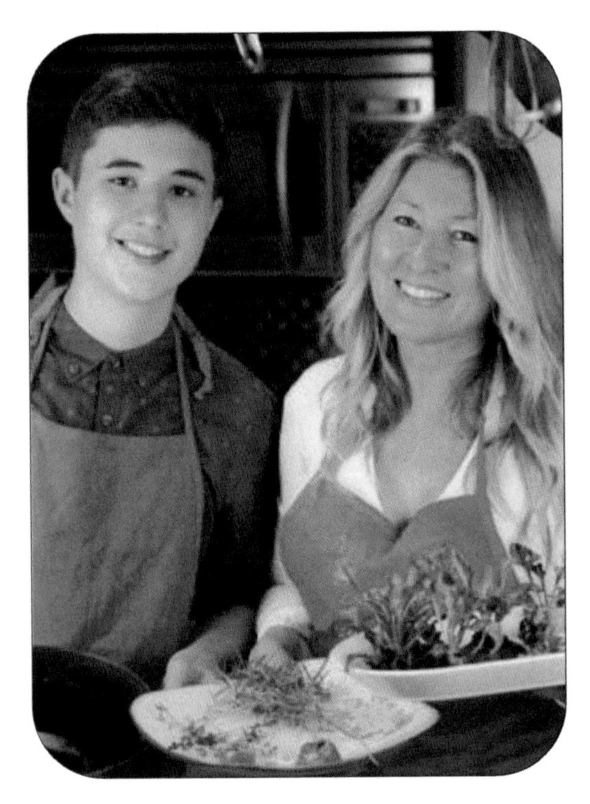

Susan Gouveia has always loved getting her hands dirty. As a child, some of her fondest memories are of helping her grandmother in the garden and cooking delicious meals from whatever was harvested from their efforts. Decades later, she has turned that love of gardening and passion for cooking into a local institution, The Society of Garden Goddesses®.

Established in 2010, The Society of Garden Goddesses® is a group of over 1,200 men and women who are interested in sustainable gardening practices. The group has grown like wildflowers—almost doubling in size from the 750 members it had on November 4, 2016. "Suddenly everyone wants to know how to grow their own food, and I'm so happy to have a forum to help them on that journey," Gouveia said. "We share tips, recipes, and lots of laughs! I wanted to take the seriousness and chore out of gardening and cooking and get people excited about experimenting with food grown in one's own garden."

More than just a group of gardeners, this is a family; a "tribe" that gets together for fun events that include: garden tour potlucks every month, Happy Gardening Hour taste and learn events at Weiss Brothers Nursery, holiday bazaars, volunteer projects, demos, classes, contests, world-renowned guest speakers, monthly guided group meditations (which are currently full with a waiting list), and much more.

A few years ago, Gouveia had two nearly fatal car accidents that clarified her life's mission. In one accident she rolled her Chevy Tahoe on the way to Lake Tahoe, and on the other she was rear ended by a drunk driver while waiting for the light to change at Alta Sierra Drive on Hwy. 49—a mere five minutes from home. "When that happened, I was so lucky to survive, and through the whole ordeal I felt that I was receiving a message," she recalled. "I was told to commit to community; that my role is to connect people and bring back that sense of community through cooking together, meditating, and networking."

Over the years, Gouveia has added more than just the gardening aspect to her repertoire of services. She is also a personal chef and has studied with chefs in Spain, Mexico, Brazil, Italy, France and Peru. Using that knowledge, along with a natural and healthy eating philosophy, Gouveia not only cooks for individuals and families looking to learn a more sustainable way of eating, she caters private parties and has also been working with schools to create sustainable fundraisers. "Instead of selling wrapping paper or candy, mass produced in a factory, we can do things that are so much more creative and locally focused," Gouveia said.

In addition, Gouveia offers cooking classes both in her gorgeous home kitchen and online through video conferencing for those who are interested but live out of the area. For the video classes, she sends a list of ingredients to the students before the class, and then walks them through a recipe. These classes can have up to 50 people and have become very popular. "People love it! Some students just need a little extra help in the kitchen or want to expand their culinary skills, and I feel honored that I get to help them with that," Gouveia said.

Never one to sit still, her newest projects have been to develop a fermentation station in her home to make dandelion wine (which tastes like early spring), an apple cider recipe that was created by Martha Washington, special herbal medicines, meads, and more. She also hosts farm tours on her property, tastings of the produce she grows and the creations she makes from her bounty, individual and couples retreats, gong therapy, and a gorgeous AirBnB rental on the Garden Goddess® Farm that leaves guests refreshed and relaxed no matter how long they stay. "This place is dedicated to teaching about sustainability," Gouveia said. "I'm trying to honor each season and appreciating the bounty of each harvest."

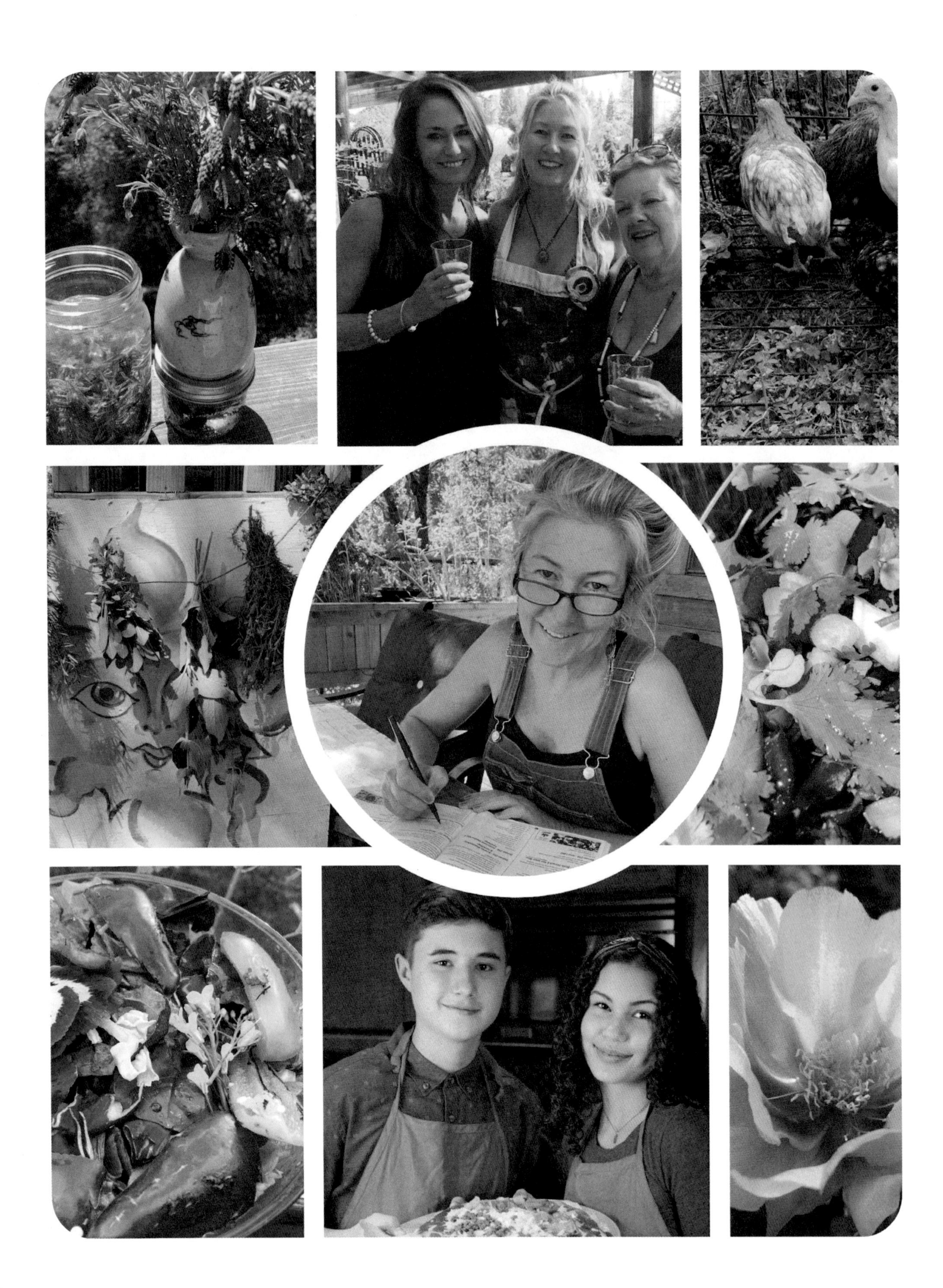

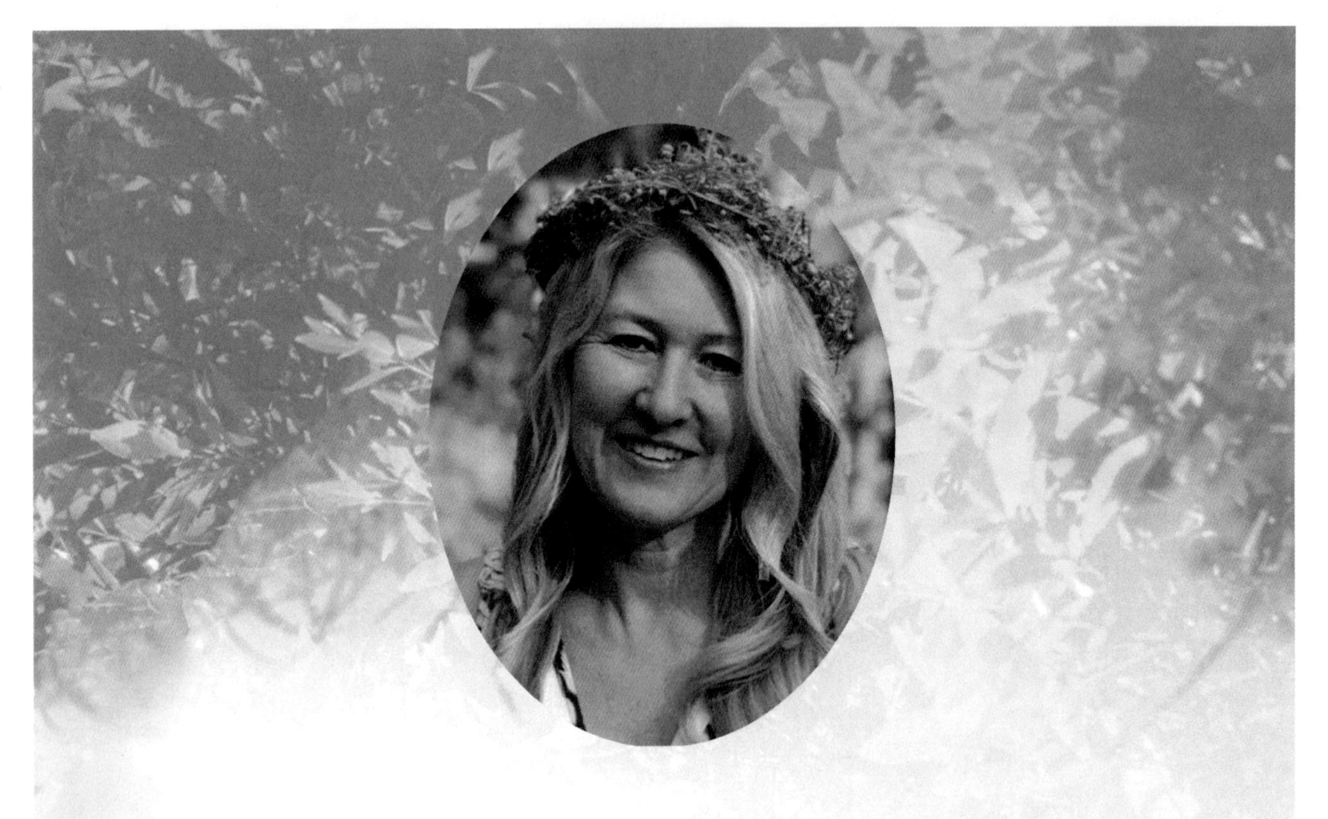

SUSAN GOUVEIA

Susan Nelson Gouveia has been passionate about foraging the land for food and medicine ever since she was a child. She began cooking family meals when her mom cut her loose in the kitchen. She rarely ever watched TV and has an on-going lust for creativity.

"When I decided to be my authentic self and go back to who I was at nine, my world changed and my tribe evolved. Today, I am living a passionate life with great friends, family, food, and creative projects."

Susan is currently a private chef and culinary teacher. She spends her days writing recipes, entertaining, homesteading, and learning new things at Garden Goddess Farm—her "university," as her son calls it.

Website: gardengoddesses.org

1

Family & Food

Susan Gouveia

"Cooking with intention, love and joy is one of the best gifts you can give to yourself, your family and community."

~ Susan Gouveia

My parents celebrate 60 years together this year. My love of food, especially as it brings family and friends together is inspired by my parents' love of healthy food. Their stories about mealtime as they were growing up reveal why.

As the eldest daughter in a family of 10, my mom remembers being frequently reminded of the expense of providing for eight hearty appetites. The goal was to "extend" every meal. She says, "Dad shopped with a keen eye for a deal and cooked to 'extend' each ingredient to a few dinners."

One-pot meals were standard, and meat was scarce, so spaghetti was flavored with watered-down tomato sauce and peppered with specks of hamburger. Stew was mostly potatoes, a couple of carrots, a stalk or two of celery, and the hunt was on for the bits of fatty meat. Other meals included: Pot of Beans—just kidney beans, and his special 'Dutch pea soup'—a sickly, green color thick enough to stand a spoon in. Cut up hot dogs in creamed corn was popular with the youngest kids. We'd alternate spaghetti and beans until, finally, they were combined for yet another meal.

Breakfast never varied: mush—cornmeal or oatmeal. Lunch was just as predictable: egg or tuna salad sandwiches, spread so thin it would rip the bread.

Mom's happiest memory of food and family was running home when the kids smelled the weekly loaves of her mom's bread, ready to come out of the oven. A fresh hot slice of bread was a favorite memory for all the kids, and was the smell that kept the kids coming back to the house.

As the eldest son in a family of seven, my dad's life-long love of fishing—especially salmon fishing in the Monterey Bay—came from a revelation that fresh salmon in no way resembled his childhood Friday salmon loaf, which tasted like cat food and was required eating or he would surely go to hell! Equally horrible were Friday fish sticks, but those, at least, he could drown in ketchup.

As a reaction to these and other family meals, my parents raised my sister and me on freshly caught fish and eggs from our own chickens. They grew fresh vegetables and fruit and, while we were on camping and fishing trips, they taught us a little about foraging and the pleasures of nature.

Writing this book has been a great way to connect with family!

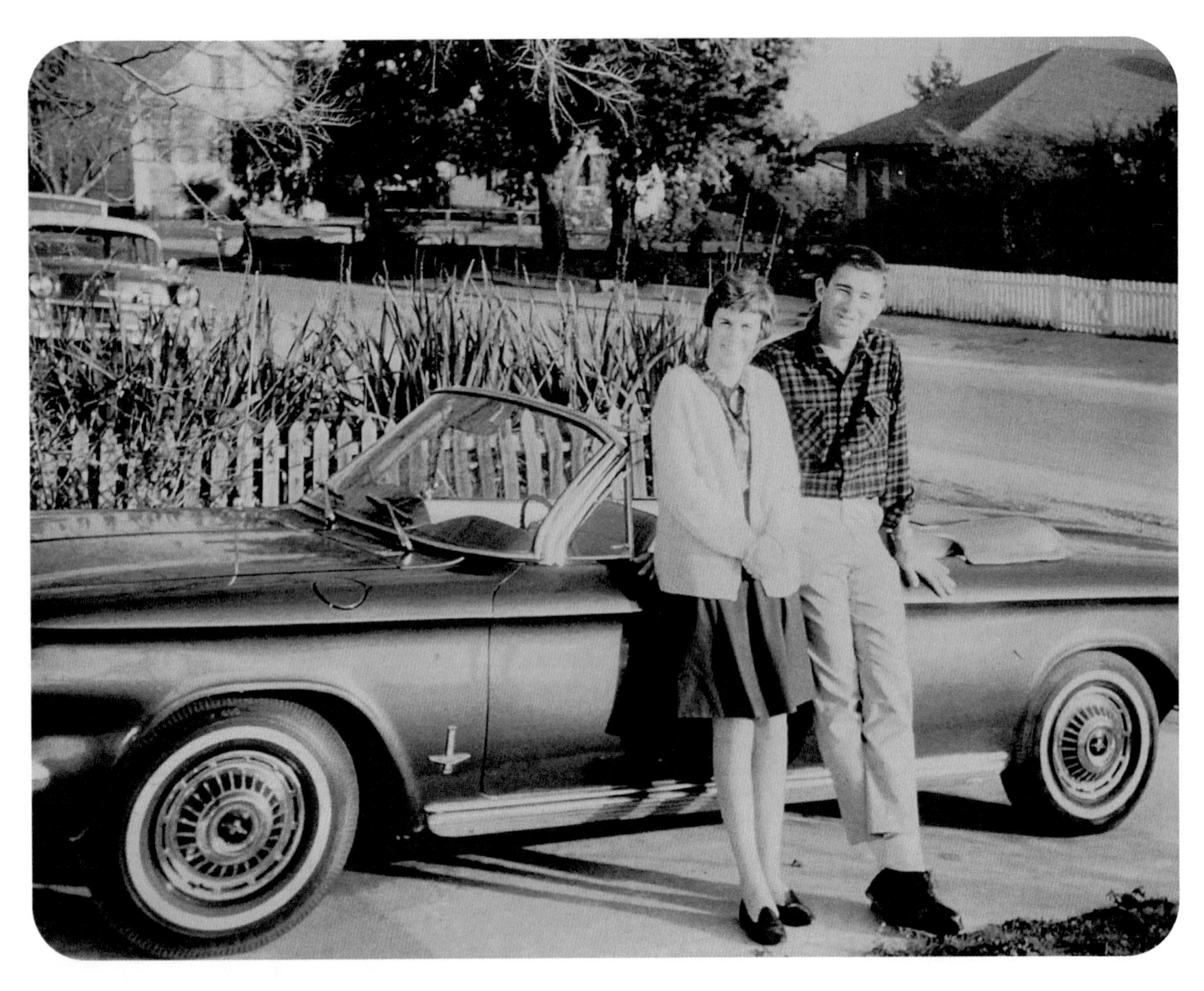

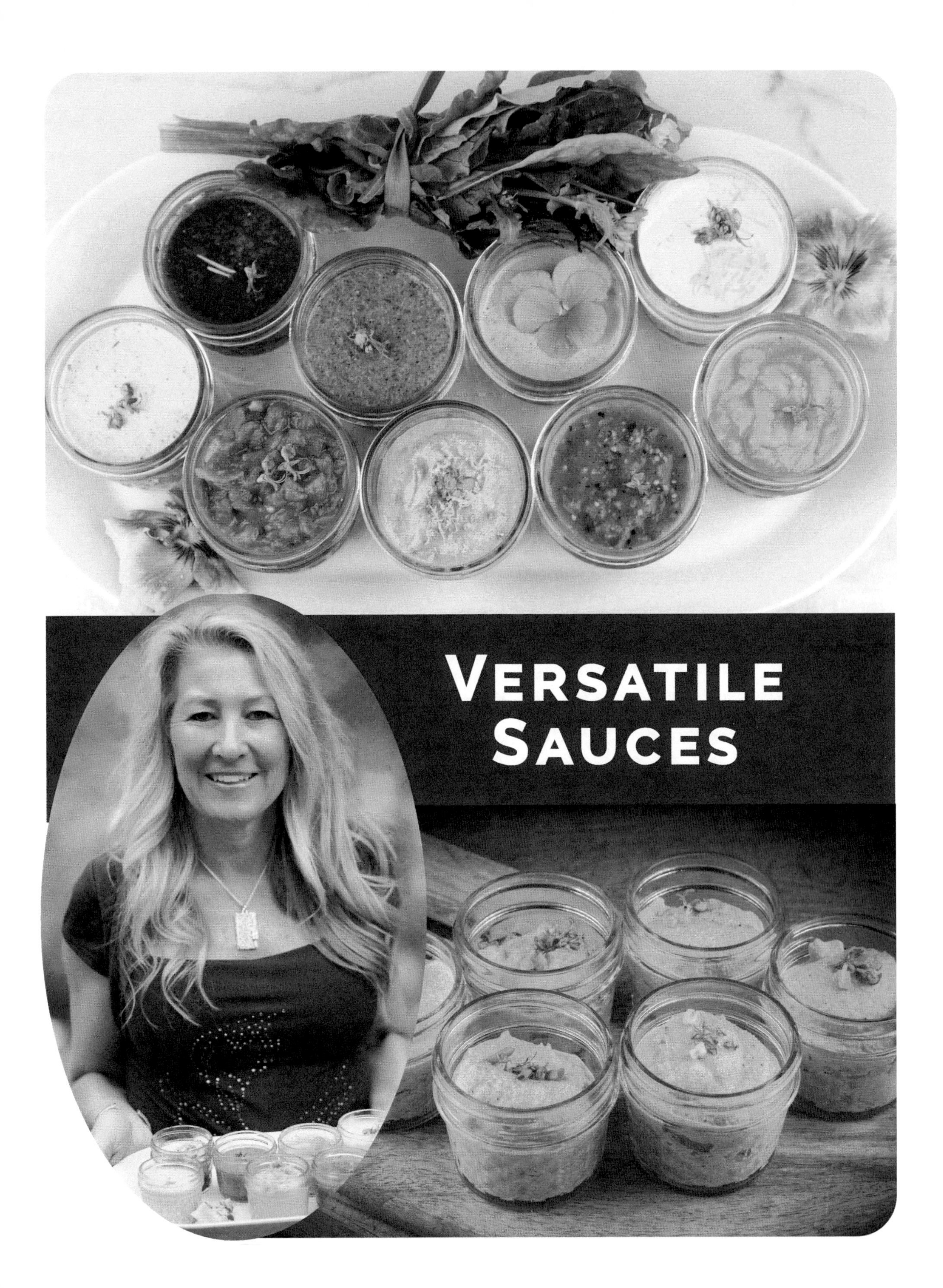

Versatile Sauces

Tantalizing Tomato Sauce

This versatile sauce can be made and canned or frozen in mason jars.

Ingredients:

- 10 medium-large tomatoes, peeled*
- 3 bell peppers
- 3 medium onions
- 3 garlic cloves
- salt, pepper, garlic powder
- balsamic vinegar
- olive or coconut oil for roasting or sautéing

* TIP: To easily peel tomatoes, freeze, and then run under hot water.

Two ways I like to prepare:

1. **Roasted**: For a sweeter flavor, roast all ingredients at 450°F until you reach the desired caramelization. Add to bowl and blend with immersion blender. This sauce will be concentrated and you may add water, broth or milk for desired consistency when using in a recipe.
2. **Pot Method**: Add onions, garlic cloves, and pepper. Sprinkle with a bit of salt to expedite caramelization. Cook until onions are translucent. Add the tomatoes and simmer for 20 minutes. Use an immersion blender to make into sauce.

Try these dishes with international flair!

- Italian Pasta & Pizza Sauce
- French Tomato Bisque: Mix sauce with cream or nut milk. Top with herbs.
- Latin Rice: Add sauce and butter (optional) to cooked rice. Garnish with cilantro.
- Spanish Tapas: Garlic Shrimp
- Southern Gumbo
- Cioppino base
- Thai Noodles: Mix with peanut butter, ginger, honey and sesame oil.
- Flavors from India: Mix with curry spices and cooked meat or veggies.

Mint Chimichuri Sauce

This versatile sauce can be made and canned or frozen in mason jars.

Ingredients:

- 1 cup firmly packed, fresh, flat-leaf parsley leaves
- 1 cup packed mint leaves
- 3 to 4 garlic cloves
- 2 T fresh oregano leaves (or substitute 2 tsp dried oregano)
- ⅓ cup extra virgin olive oil
- 2 T red wine vinegar
- ½ tsp sea salt
- ⅛ - ¼ tsp freshly ground black pepper
- ¼ tsp red pepper flakes or thinly sliced ½ of Serrano pepper

To Prepare:

Finely chop the parsley, fresh oregano, and garlic (or process in a food processor for several pulses). Place in a small bowl. Stir in the olive oil, vinegar, salt, pepper, and red pepper flakes/chili. Adjust seasonings. Serve immediately or refrigerate. If chilled, return to room temperature before serving. Keeps for a week or two.

This sauce is great for:

- Salad dressing. Add sour cream or mayonnaise for a creamier texture.
- Marinate tofu, lamb or beef. Save some to pour on after grilling.
- Use on roasted chicken.
- Dipping sauce for bread.
- Make stuffed eggs. Mix hard-boiled egg yolks with sauce and a bit of mayo and stuff into egg whites. Great appetizer or salad garnish.
- Mix with your choice of shredded cheese and add to favorite pasta.

Susan's Peanut Sauce

The secret to this sauce is adding caramelized onions!

Ingredients:

- 1 T red curry paste
- 1 tsp sesame oil
- 1 C natural peanut butter, smooth or chunky
- ¼ C honey
- 1 T soy sauce, Bragg's, or coconut liquid aminos
- 3 T lime juice or apple cider vinegar
- ⅓ C caramelized white onions
- 1 T grated or ½ tsp powdered ginger
- 1 garlic clove
- salt to taste
- ½ C or more water to create desired consistency

Blend in food processor. Season to taste.

This sauce is great for:

- Gado Gado Indonesian rice bowls.
- Dipping sauce for meat skewers.
- Mix sauce with coconut milk, spicy chili pepper, and veggies for a peanut curry soup.
- **Pad Thai style noodles**: Cook up some rice noodles, add some shredded cabbage, carrot, or bean sprouts. Stir in peanut sauce and garnish with fresh squeezed lime, crushed peanuts and fresh cilantro, green onion or parsley.
- **Lettuce wraps**: Make a tray of cut veggies and meat for guests to choose from. Use romaine, iceberg, butter lettuce or cabbage leaves and drizzle with sauce. Guests add their desired ingredients.
- **Thai inspired tacos:** Fill tortillas with meat or tofu. Add herbs, shredded cabbage, diced onions and chopped veggies. Top with sauce.

Goddess Avocado Chutney

Make extra and freeze in little 4 oz. mason jars for a quick sauce, snack or dip.

Ingredients:

- 4 large ripe avocados
- 3 green onions
- 1-2 garlic cloves
- handful of cilantro
- 1 lemon, zested and juiced
- 1 small green pepper, mild or spicy
- ¼ C of cottage cheese, sour cream or Greek plain yogurt, (or dairy free alternative)
- 1-2 T of liquid aminos. (I like coconut aminos for a bit of sweetness.)
- salt, pepper and garlic powder to taste
- ¼ C to 1 C water. Add slowly for desired consistency.

Blend all ingredients in food processor and season to taste.

This sauce is great for:

- Salad Dressing: Blend with a few anchovies for an Avocado Caesar Salad.
- Cabbage Salad: Use as an alternative to mayonnaise in a coleslaw.
- Tacos
- Dipping Sauce for spring rolls
- Baked Potatoes: Use instead of butter.
- Rice or rice noodles can be topped with it. Add green scallion and pine nuts.

Cashew "Cheese" Sauce

Ingredients:

- 2 C cashews (soak 2 hours in water)
- 3 T lemon juice
- 2-4 C water
- ¼ C nutritional yeast
- ½ tsp paprika
- 1 tsp garlic powder or 1 garlic clove
- 1 tsp onion powder
- ½ tsp chili powder
- 1 tsp salt
- 1-2 tsp Sriracha sauce
- ½ tsp turmeric

Mix all ingredients in a food processor or blender. Add water a little at a time until desired consistency. When using as a "cheese" make thicker. For dressings make thinner.

Fun uses:

- Tastes great as a "cheese" on pizza when baked.
- Vegan Nachos: drizzle on corn tortilla chips and add green onion, olives, colorful peppers and refried beans. Heat in oven if desired.
- Top tacos, instead of sour cream.
- Top macaroni noodles for a tasty Mac 'n "Cheese".

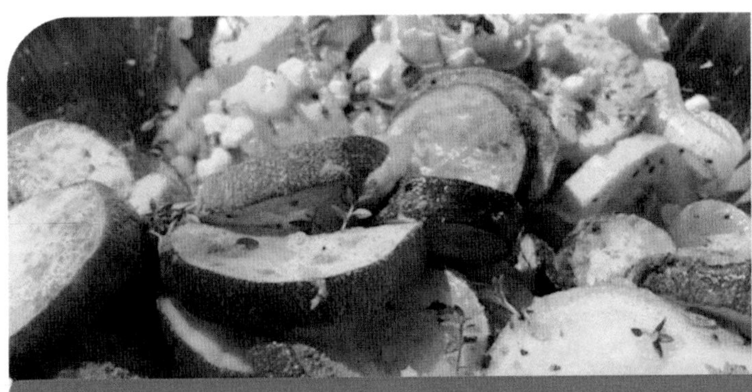
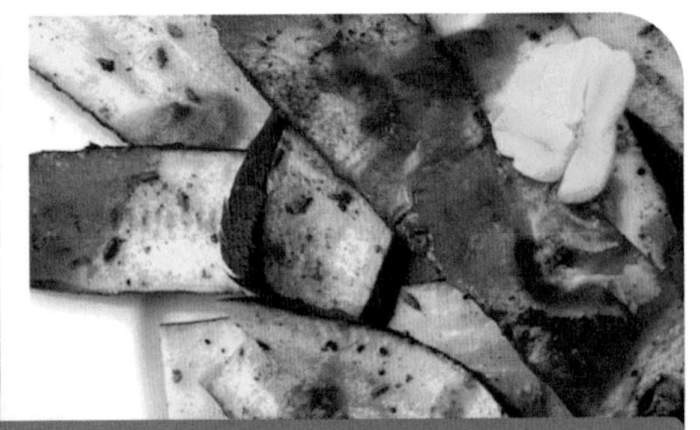

ZUCCHINI!

Creative ways to enjoy Squash

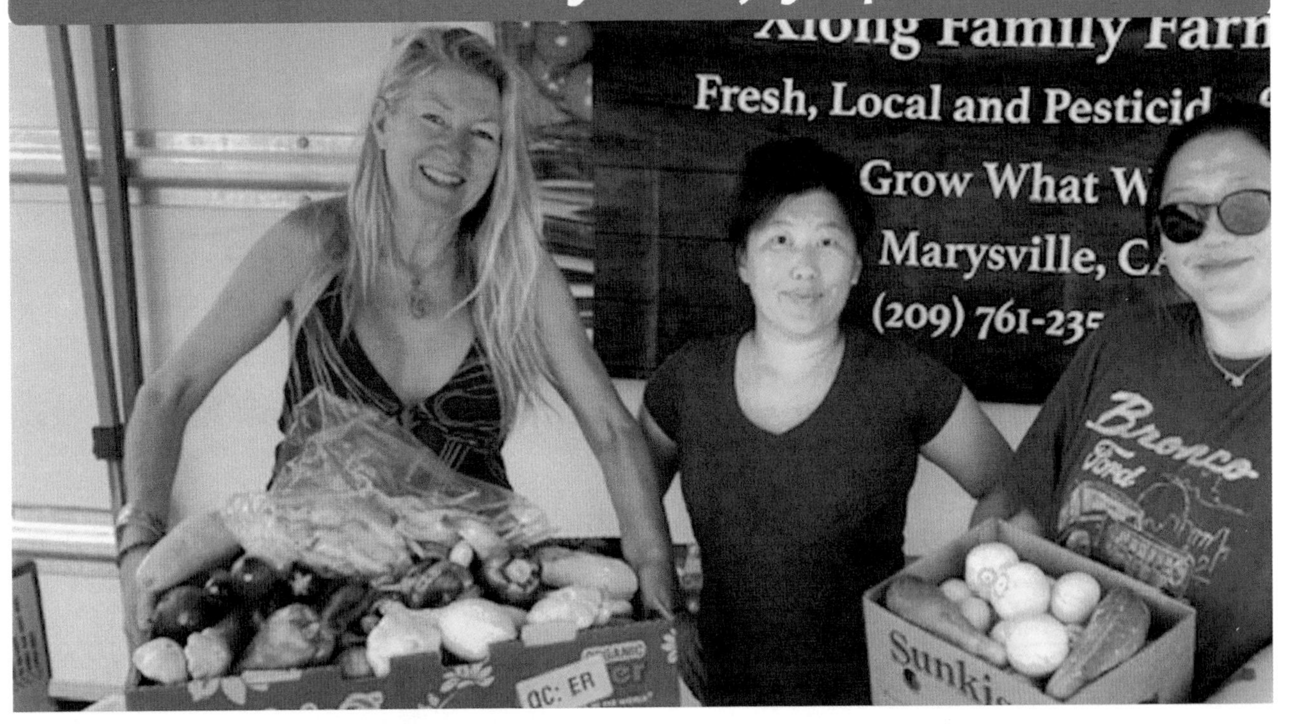

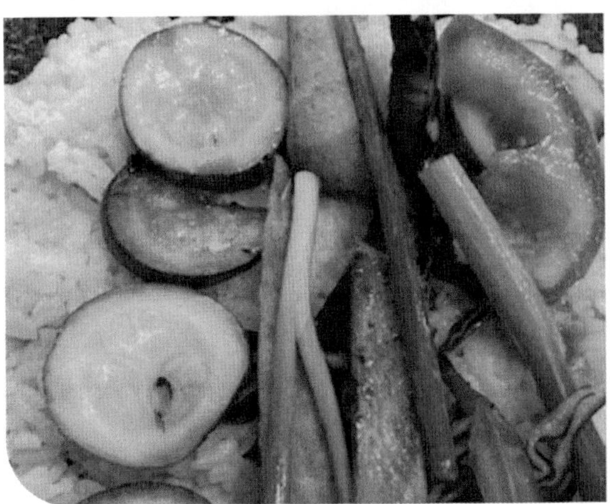
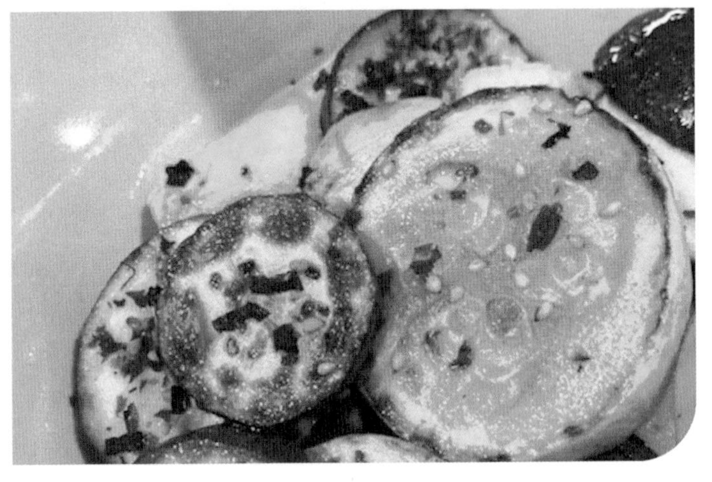

Zucchini & Mint Summer Salad

Ingredients:

- 3 medium zucchini
- 4 sprigs of mint
- 1 lemon
- 2 T extra-virgin olive oil
- Salt to taste

To Prepare:

Wash, trim and slice zucchini thinly. I like to use a mandolin.

Layer zucchini slices onto a serving platter.

Take mint leaves off their stems and stack in a layer. Roll the leaves lengthwise and cut into thin ribbons. Sprinkle on top of zucchini.

Zest the lemon over the zucchini. Once you have most of the zest, cut the lemon in half and squeeze the juice over the zucchini.

Drizzle zucchini with olive oil and sprinkle with a finishing salt to taste.

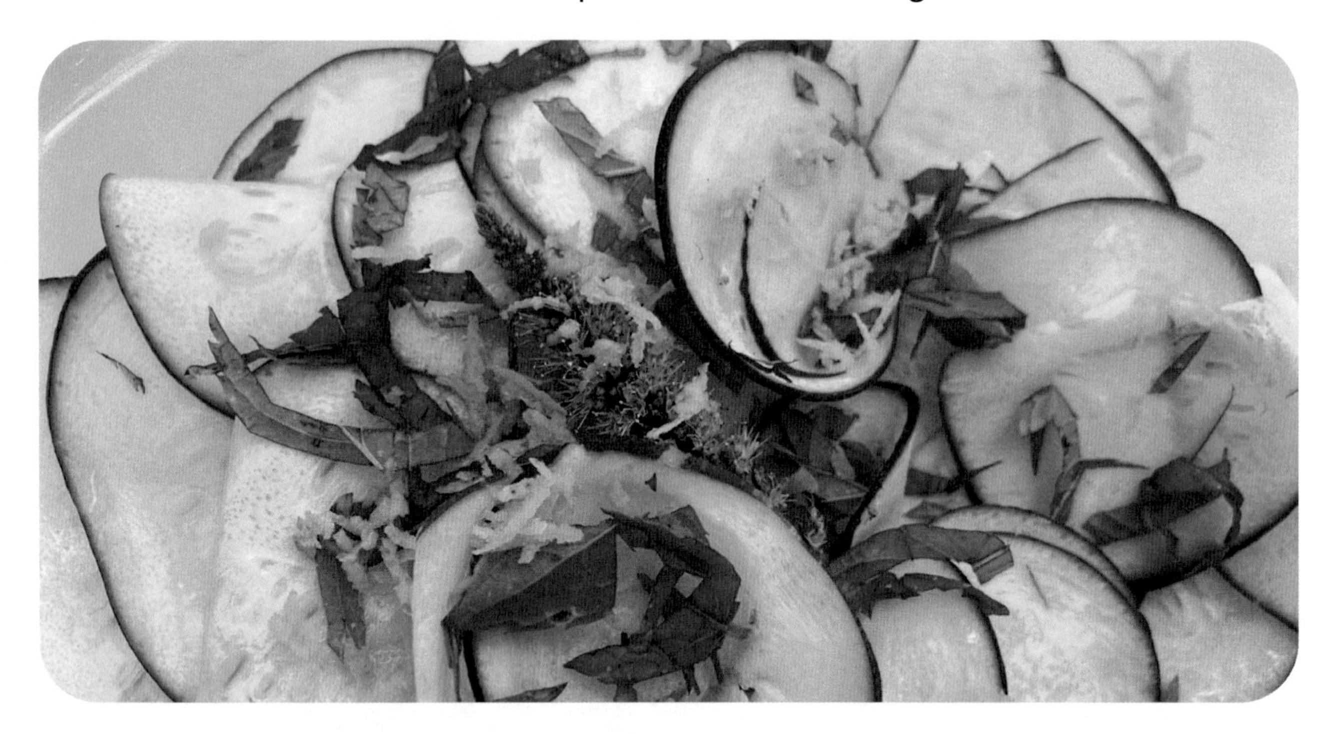

Zucchini & Sweet Potato Pancakes

Ingredients:

- 2 C grated zucchini
- 1 C grated sweet potato
- ½ tsp salt
- 3 large eggs
- ¾ C grated cheese, your choice
- 3 tsp finely chopped parsley
- 3 tsp finely chopped scallion
- ¼ C chickpea flour
- ¼ tsp freshly ground black pepper
- 2 T unsalted butter

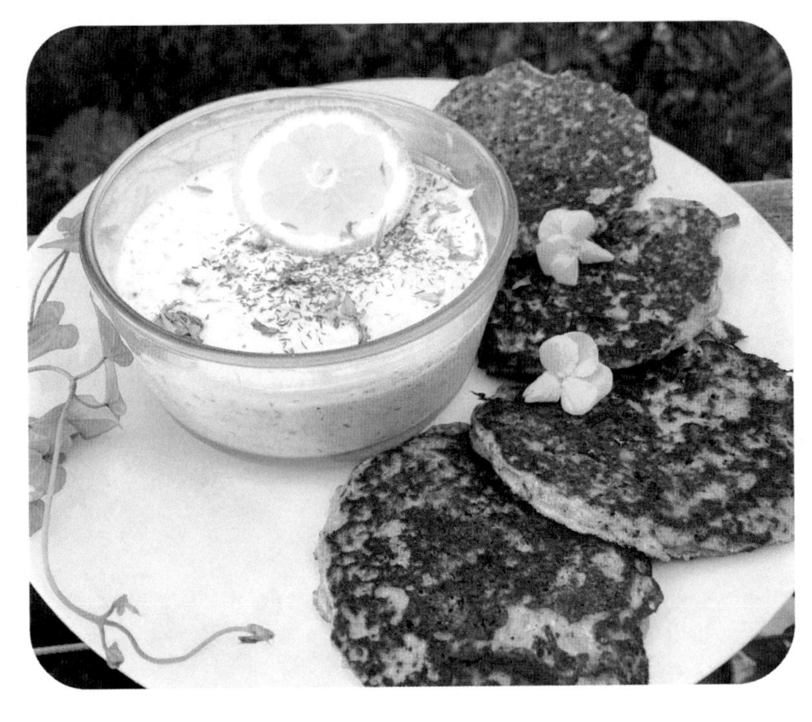

To Prepare:

Put the shredded zucchini in a colander and mix with the salt. Cover and let drain for about 30 minutes. Reserve the liquid to use in a salad dressing.

In a mixing bowl, combine the zucchini and the sweet potato with the beaten eggs, cheese, herbs, flour, and pepper.

Heat butter in a large skillet or griddle over medium heat. Spoon a few tablespoons of the zucchini batter into the skillet for each pancake and cook until browned on the bottom. Turn and cook until browned on the other side.

Serve as an appetizer with sweet or savory dip.

Yogurt dill sauce or pesto go great with this dish!

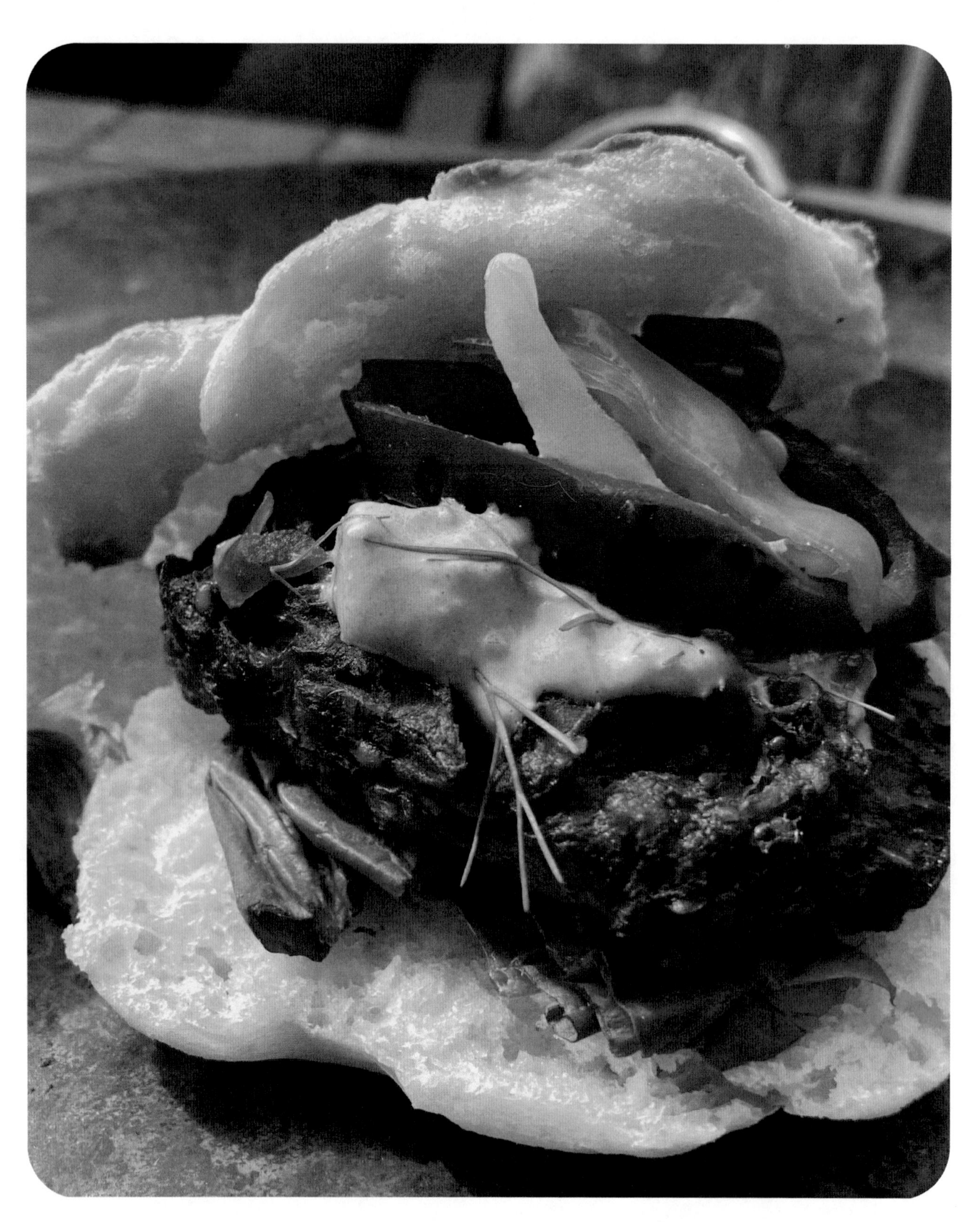

Zucchini Quinoa Sliders

For Dill Dipping Sauce:

- ½ C Greek yogurt or sour cream
- 2 tsp freshly squeezed lemon juice
- ½ tsp lemon zest
- 1 – 2 tsp chopped fresh dill
- 1 tsp honey
- sea salt to taste

For Sliders:

- 3 medium zucchini, shredded (about 4 cups)
  Place in colander & sprinkle with salt to remove the excess water.
- 3-4 eggs
- 1 small yellow onion, grated
- 1 C cooked quinoa
- ¾ C panko breadcrumbs
- 2 T grated Parmesan cheese
- ¼ – ½ tsp chipotle powder
- ½ tsp paprika
- ⅓ C parsley chopped finely
- ¼ C green onion
- ½ tsp sea salt or to taste
- freshly ground black pepper, to taste
- 3 T olive oil, or more as needed
- butter

To Prepare Dill Dipping Sauce:

Combine all ingredients in a small bowl. Whisk to blend. Season with salt to taste.

To Prepare Sliders:

Add eggs to a large bowl and beat lightly. Add the rest of the ingredients and stir until well combined.

Add the oil/butter to a griddle, or 10-inch skillet and heat over medium heat. Add approximately ¼ C of the slider mixture to the skillet.

Cook until golden around the edges and set, 3-4 minutes. Flip and cook 3-4 minutes more, or until golden all over. Transfer to a paper towel-lined dish to drain.

Serve with the dipping sauce. Place sliders on garlic toasts, buns or lettuce leaves.

Chilled Summer Squash Soup

Ingredients:

- 1 medium onion, coarsely chopped
- 1 clove garlic
- 1 T olive oil
- 1 tsp butter
- ½ tsp salt to taste
- 4 medium zucchinis
- 3 to 4 C vegetable broth
- ½ C coconut milk
- black pepper, freshly ground

To Prepare:

Trim and chop the zucchini, discard the ends. Heat a medium pot over medium heat. Add oil, butter, garlic and onions. Cook until translucent and tender, approximately 5 minutes, stirring occasionally,

Add zucchini and broth to the onions/garlic. Bring to a boil. Reduce the heat immediately after boiling and maintain a steady simmer until zucchini is very tender, about 15-20 minutes.

Once the zucchini is cooked, turn off heat. Use an immersion blender to make into a creamy soup. Serve warm or chilled with a selection of toppings for your guests.

Garnish Options: Coarsely chopped fresh dill, cilantro, parsley or green onion, colorful peppers, (mild or spicy), turmeric, paprika, or beet powder, bacon or salmon

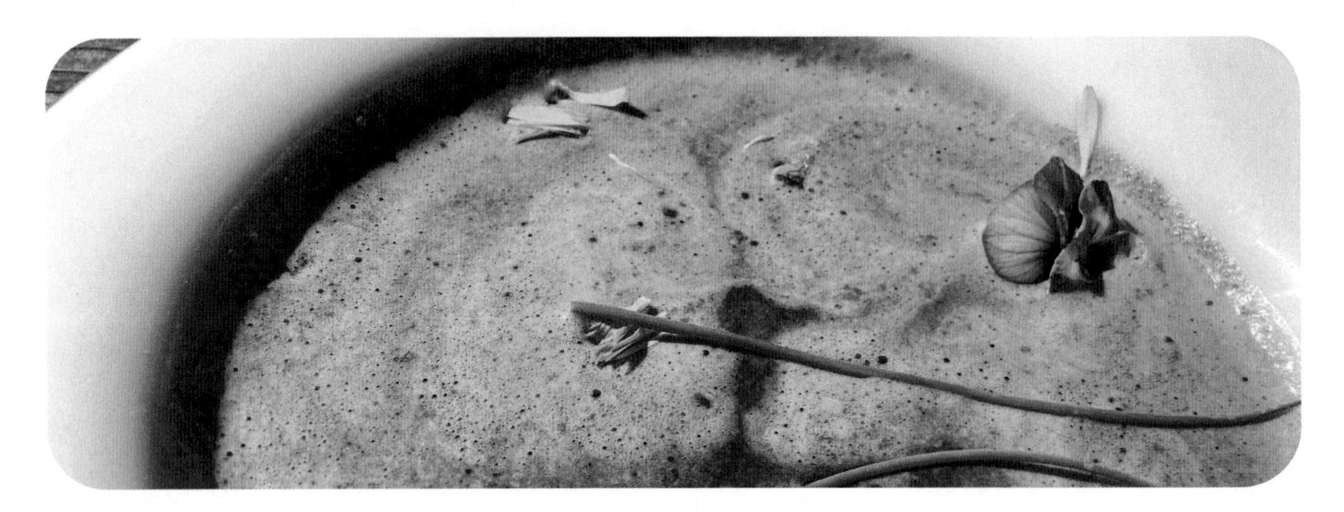

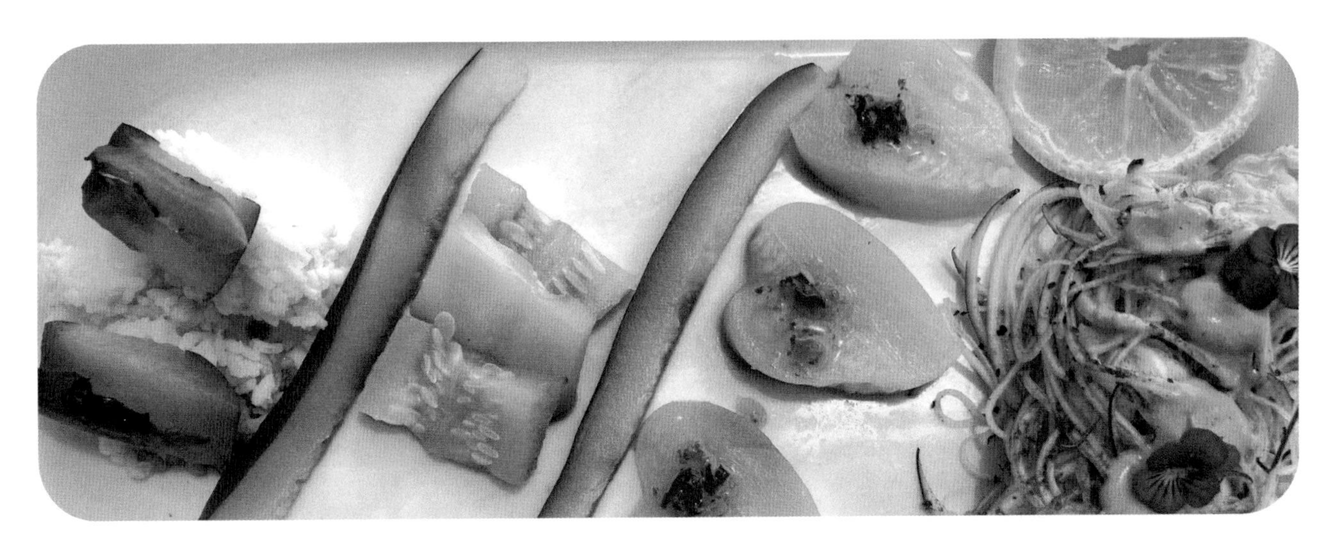

Roasted Pepper Zucchini Nigiri

Ingredients:

- 1 medium zucchini
- 1 T Braggs liquid aminos or coconut aminos
- 1 T maple syrup
- ½ tsp sriracha sauce
- 1 tsp rice vinegar
- 1 to 2 C cooked sushi rice
- 1 or 2 red, yellow, purple or orange pepper

To Prepare:

Trim zucchini and slice lengthwise to desired thickness. If you are trying to replicate fish, peel green skin off. Cut in rectangular pieces and steam cook until pieces are soft and translucent. Remove zucchini from heat and cool on a serving dish

Meanwhile roast peppers over flame until charred. Next, mix the marinade and pour desired amount over zucchini pieces. Make sushi rice balls to lay the zucchini and a slice of roasted pepper on. (When squishing the rice in your hand to make the shapes to lay veggies on, it's easier if you have a bowl of water to rinse your hands in so rice does not stick to you.)

Serve nigiri or sashimi style. Garnished of course! Ginger, lemon slices and green onion are a good choice!

Spicy Zucchini Boats

Ingredients:

- 4 medium zucchinis
- 1 T olive oil
- 5 shallots, diced
- ½ C of cooked bacon or sausage
- 1 red, yellow, or green bell pepper, diced
- ½ tsp garlic powder
- ½-1 tsp of Sriracha sauce
- ¼ C bread crumbs
- salt & pepper to taste
- ¼ sliced green onion
- ½ C shredded, flavorful cheeses of your choice
- sour cream or Greek yogurt for garnish

To Prepare:

Preheat the oven to 375°F. Cut off the stem end of the zucchinis and slice them in half lengthwise. With a spoon or melon baller, scoop out just the pulpy center that contains the seeds. Dice and put aside for the filling.

Place the zucchini halves, cut-side down, on a parchment paper-lined baking sheet. Bake for 15 minutes or until just slightly softened.

While the zucchini are baking, in a sauté pan, heat the olive oil over medium heat. Add the shallots, bell pepper, and diced zucchini. Sauté until they are softened, about 5 minutes. Remove pan from heat. Sprinkle mixture with garlic powder. Stir in the rest of the ingredients. Season mixture with salt and pepper.

Remove the zucchini from the oven and turn them over on the sheet pan so they are cut-side up. Divide the veggie and meat mixture between the zucchini halves, spooning it into the carved-out channel where the seeds were removed.

Return the zucchini to the oven and cook for 10 minutes or until cheese is melted. Remove the zucchini from the oven, sprinkle each boat with garnish and serve with sour cream or Greek yogurt. A great brunch item served with eggs!

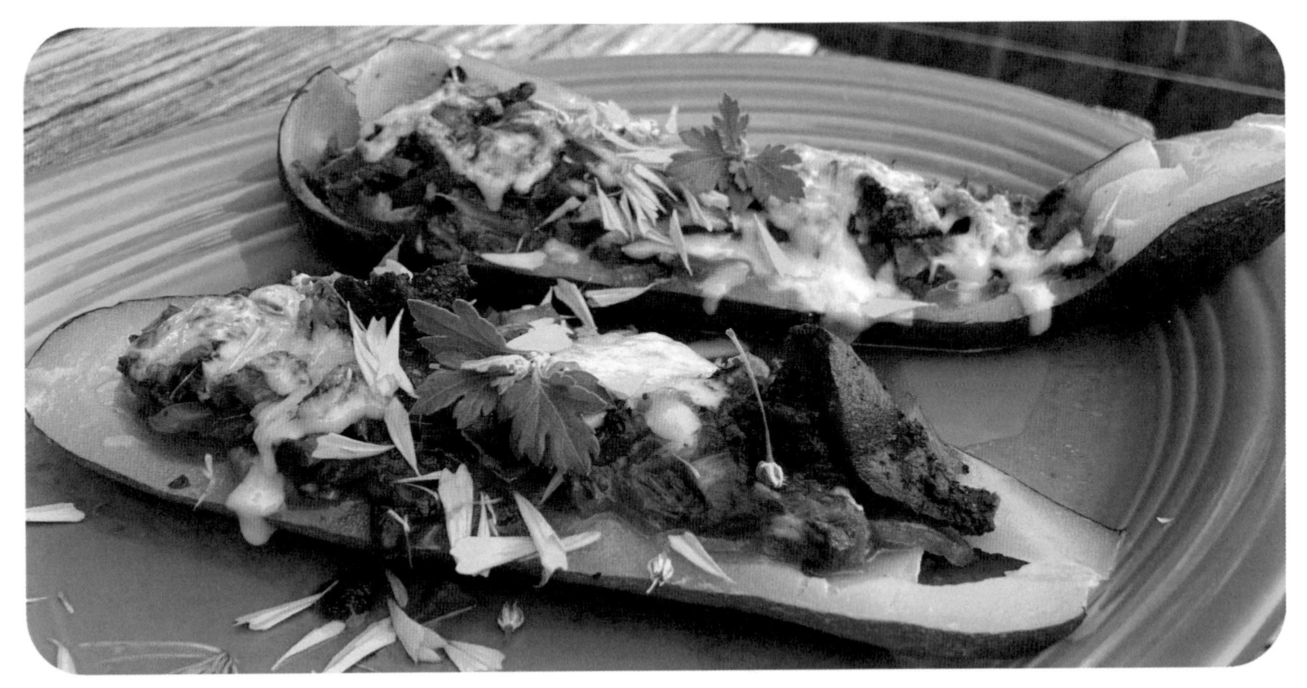

Spicy Zucchini Boats

Zucchini Crust Pizza

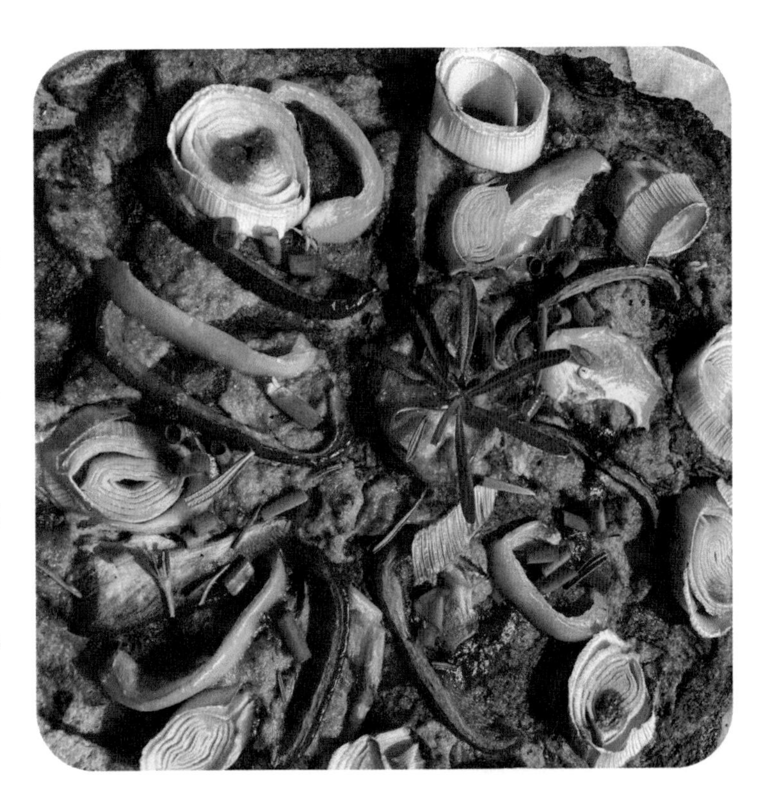

To Prepare:

Use the squash pancake (pg. 11) or cracker recipe (pg. 22) for crust.

Bake at 400°F until half-way done. Flip crust if needed.

Add sauce, cheese, and toppings as desired.

Place back in oven until cheese is melted and toppings are cooked.

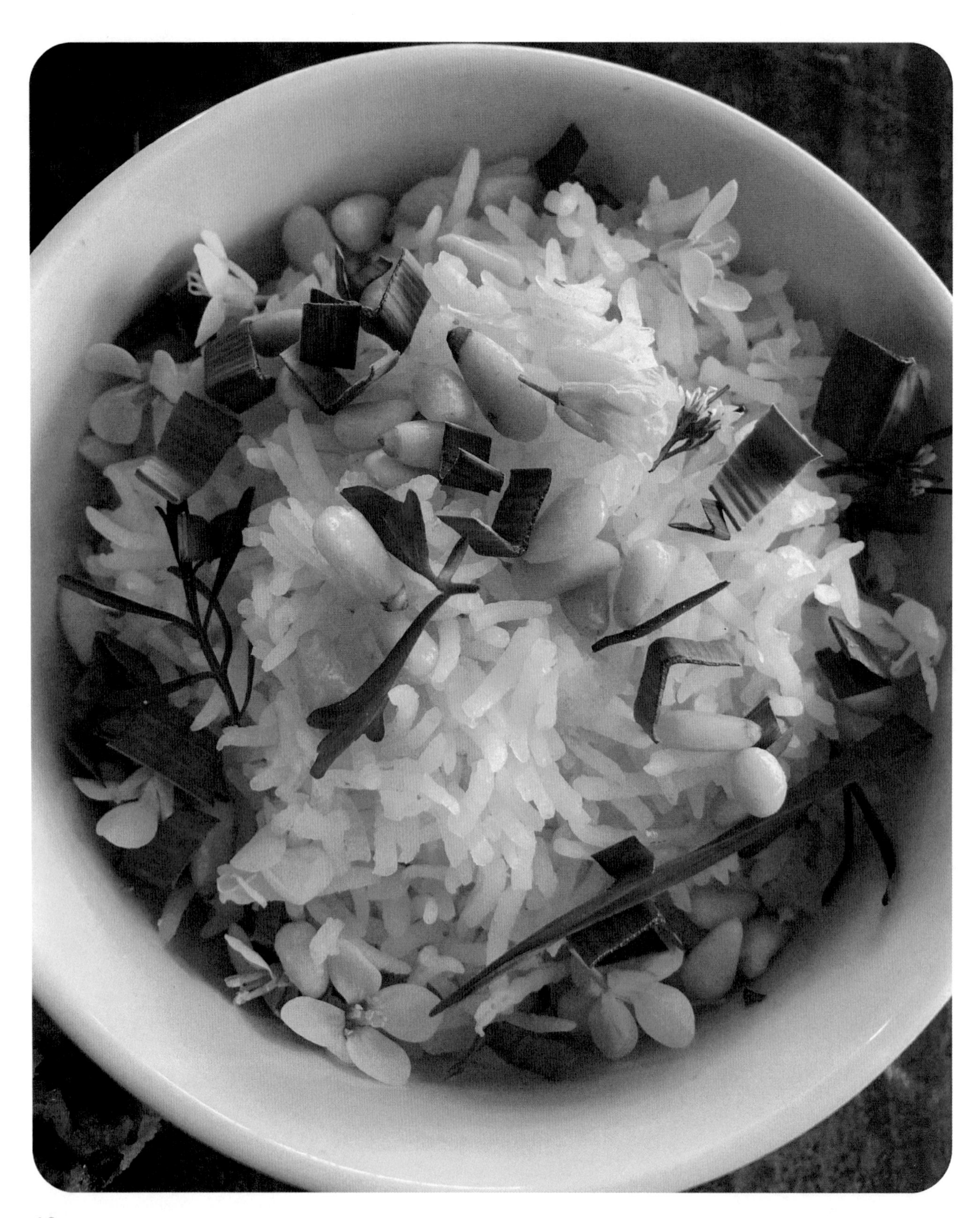

Lemon Zucchini Easy "Risotto"

Ingredients:

- 2 C of short grained rice
- ¼ C butter
- 1 C of shredded zucchini/squash
- ¼ tsp turmeric
- 1 tsp garlic powder
- 1 lemon, zested & juiced
- ½ C of parsley chopped,
- ½ C Parmesan cheese (optional)
- ¼ C shredded carrots (optional)

To Prepare:

Cook rice according to the directions and add the butter, turmeric, garlic powder and half of the parsley.

When cooked, remove lid and fluff rice with a fork, while adding the shredded zucchini/squash and optional cheese.

Put lid back on to allow the squash to steam with the remaining heat.

Before serving, season to taste with the remaining parsley, shredded carrots, fresh lemon zest and juice, salt and pepper.

Zucchini “Noodles” with Peanut Sauce

Ingredients:

- 1 large zucchini
- peanut sauce (see page 6)
- chopped cilantro for garnish

To Prepare:

Spiralize zucchini into noodles, or grate for a shorter version. Use the noodles raw or sauté in sesame oil.

Serve with peanut sauce and chopped cilantro.

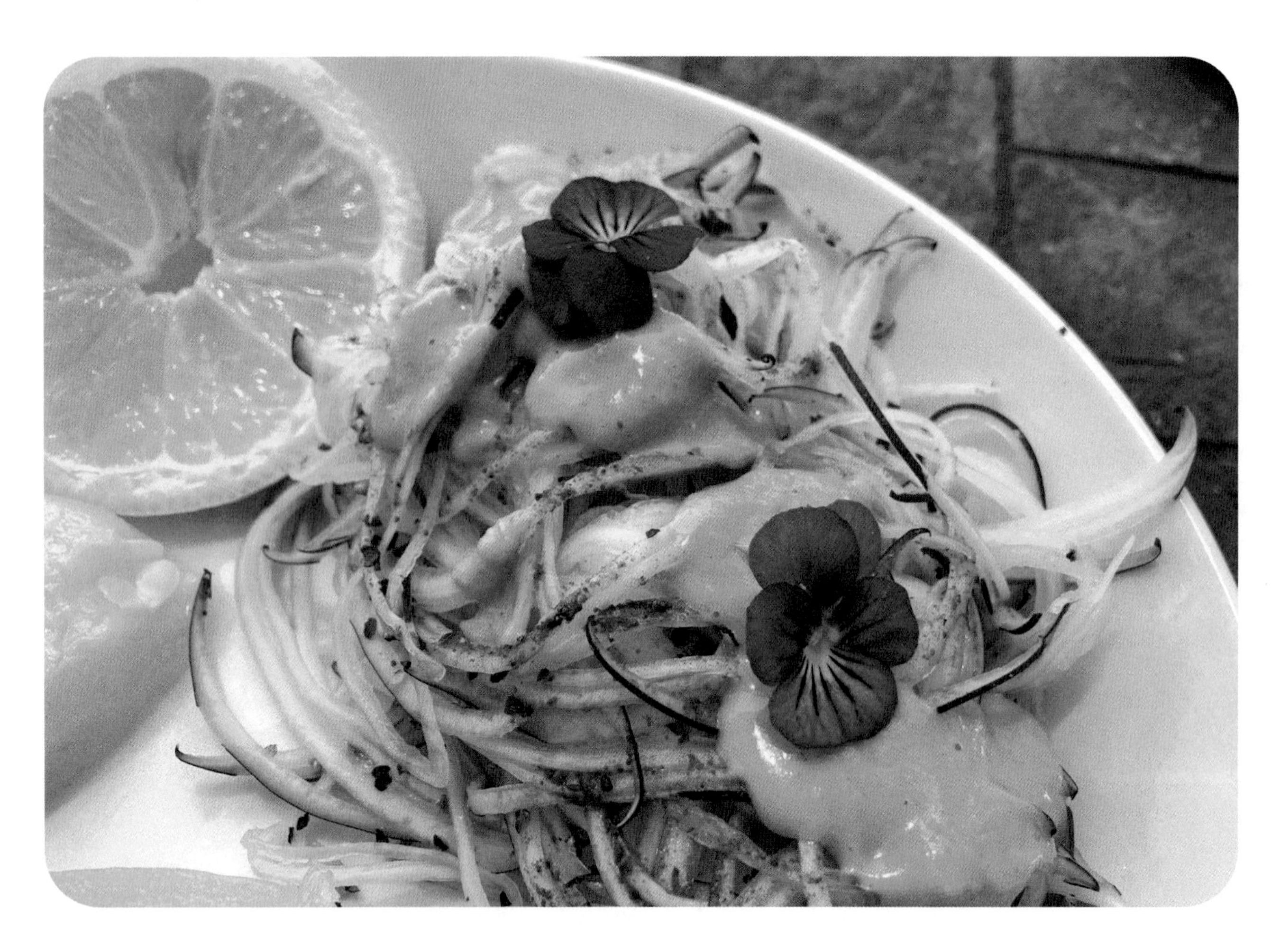

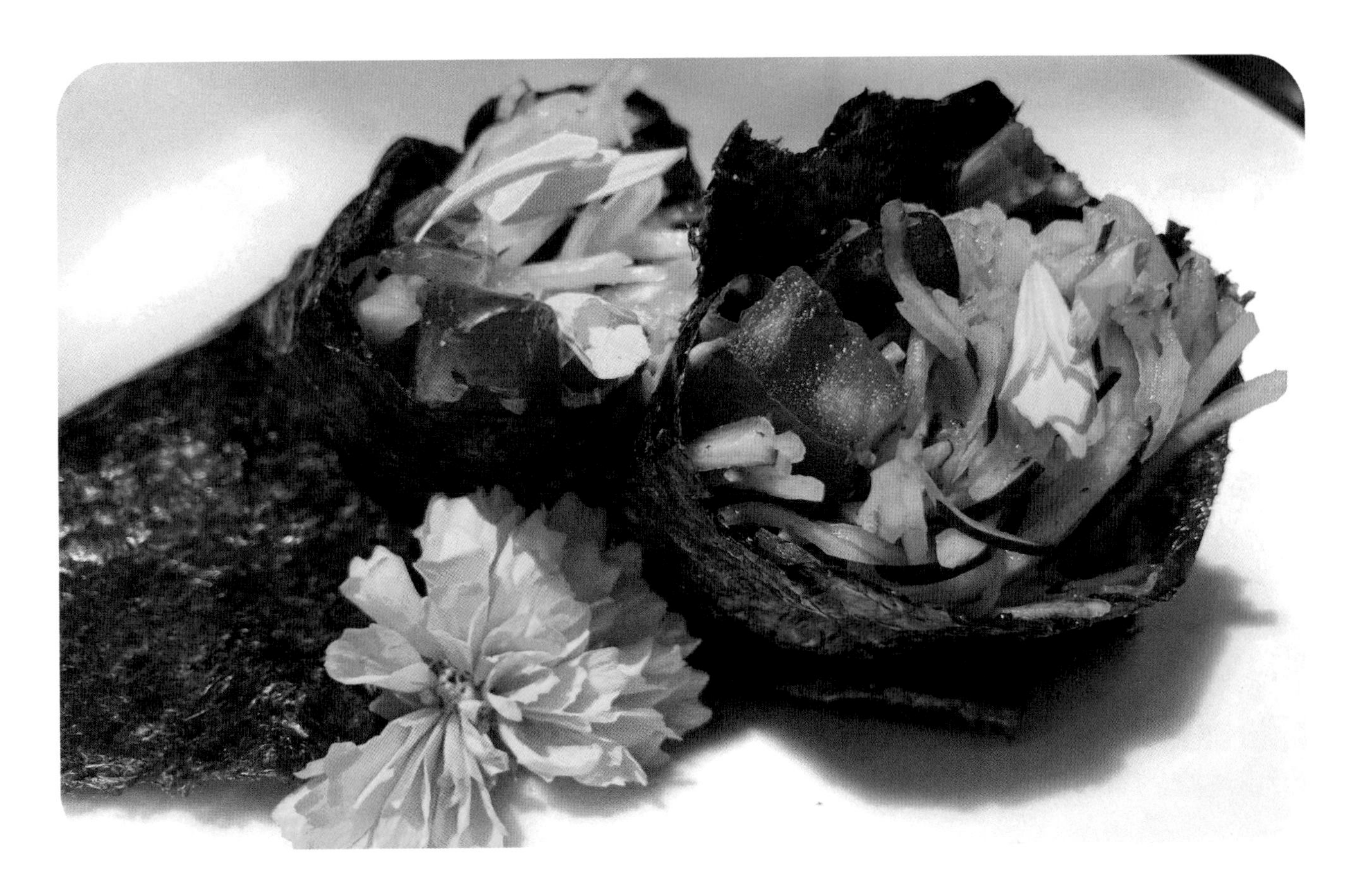

Zucchini Nori Wraps

For a guest-friendly lunch or dinner, supply the seaweed sheets, rice, sauces, and assorted veggies. Roll your own Nori Wrap!

Ingredients:

- Nori sheets (seaweed)
- Assorted veggie platter with zoodles or shredded squash, grated carrot, shredded lettuce, shredded purple cabbage, radish, and avocado
- Sushi rice
- Assorted sauce ideas: Peanut, pesto or avocado ranch

To Prepare:

Spread nori sheet with rice, veggies of your choice. Roll up and cut to desired size. Serve with sauce of your choice.

Zucchini Easy "Paté"

Ingredients:

- 1 C zucchini, trimmed and cubed
- 2 cloves garlic, minced
- ½ C red, white or yellow sweet onion, thinly sliced
- 2 T chickpea miso
- 1 T butter and/or olive oil
- balsamic vinegar, a splash
- pinch of salt

To Prepare:

Steam squash until soft. Carmelize onions by sauteeing in 1 T butter/olive oil for 10-15 minutes, being careful not to burn. Add the garlic. Add a bit of salt to "sweat out" the bitterness. When carmelized, sprinkle with a bit of balsamic vinegar and cook for another minute.

Blend all ingredients in a food processor until smooth. Chill in a mold or small bowl until firm. Serve with sundried squash crackers, veggies or garlic toasts.

Sundried Zucchini Crackers

Ingredients:

- 1 C zucchini pulp from juicing
- ⅓ sunflower seeds
- 2 T flax seed
- 1 T green onion, parsley or dill
- spices to taste: salt, pepper, garlic or onion powder, turmeric, paprika, and curry powder work well.

To Prepare:

Mix all ingredients together for a chunkier cracker or blend together in a food processor for a smoother cracker.

Spread mixture on parchment paper and dry in the sun or a dehydrator. Flip, if needed, to cook the other side until crispy. Break into pieces and serve with your favorite dip.

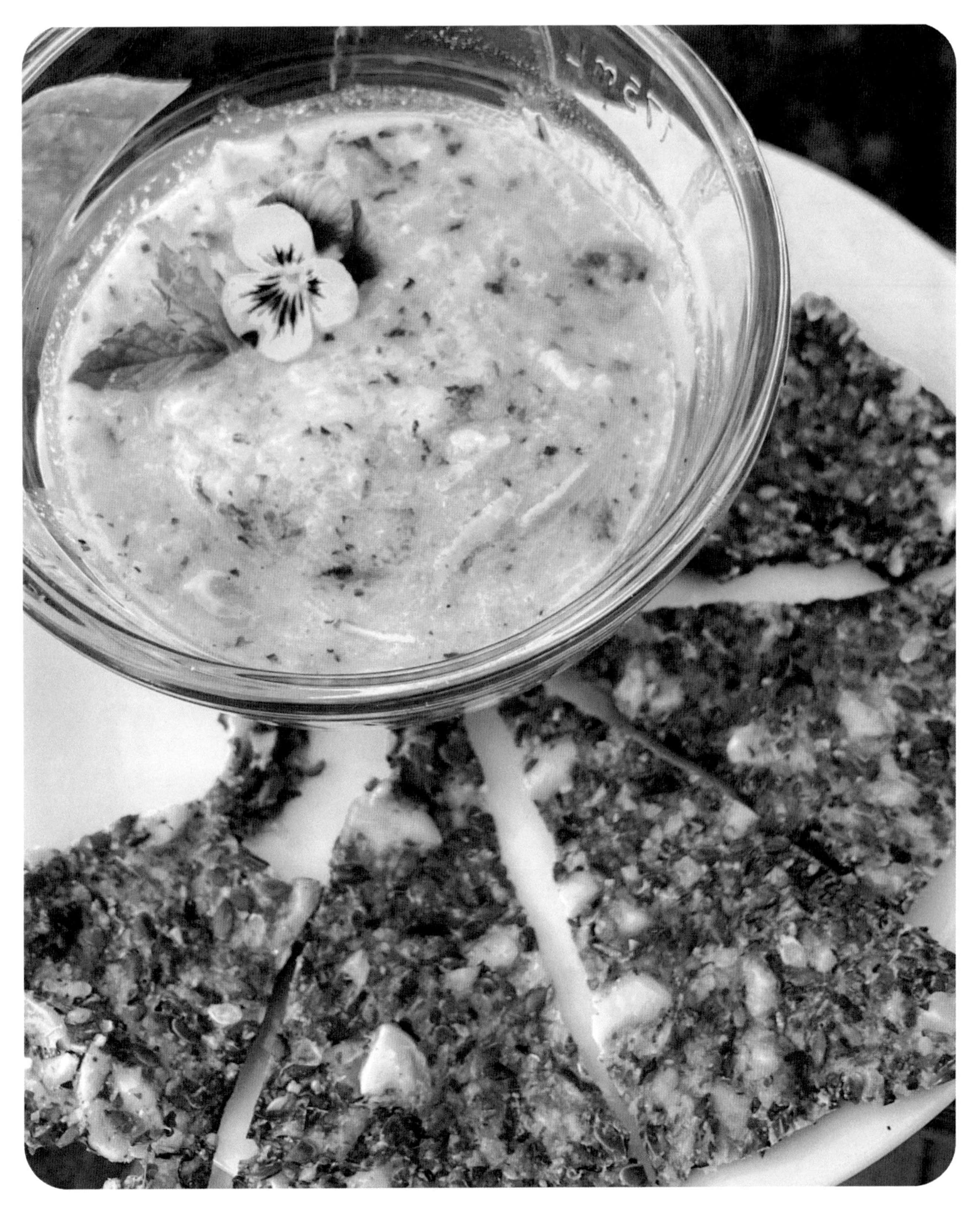

Breakfast Nest

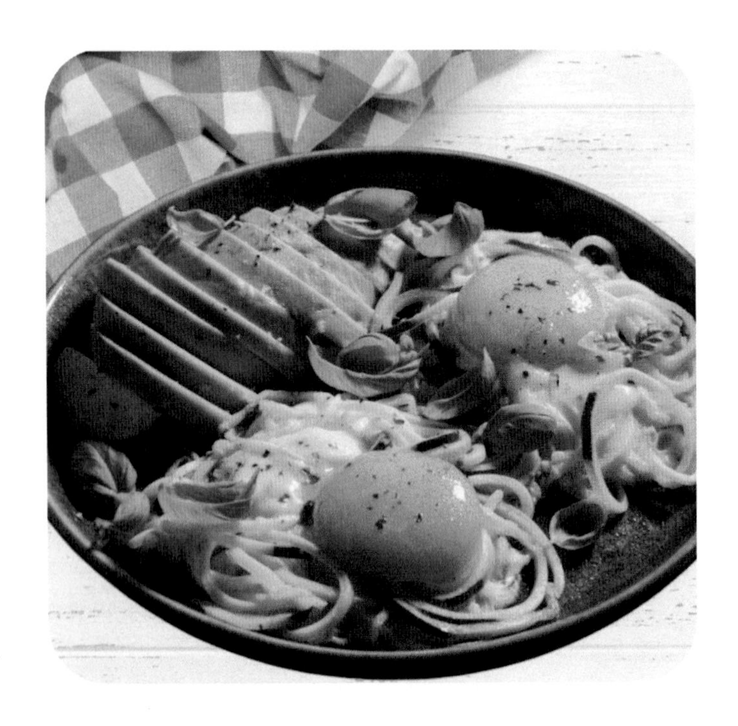

To Prepare:

Spiralize or grate a pile of squash noodles (1-2 cups) and place in a heated, buttered pan.

Make a "nest" in the noodles and crack an egg or two into it. Season with salt, pepper, garlic powder, and hot sauce, if desired.

Add 2 T of water to pan and cover. Steam for 3 minutes or until egg is done to your liking.

Heavenly Juice: Zucchini & Fruit

To Prepare:

Do you have a juicer?

Zucchini is very juicy and tastes great juiced with pineapple, apples, peaches, plums, melons and more!

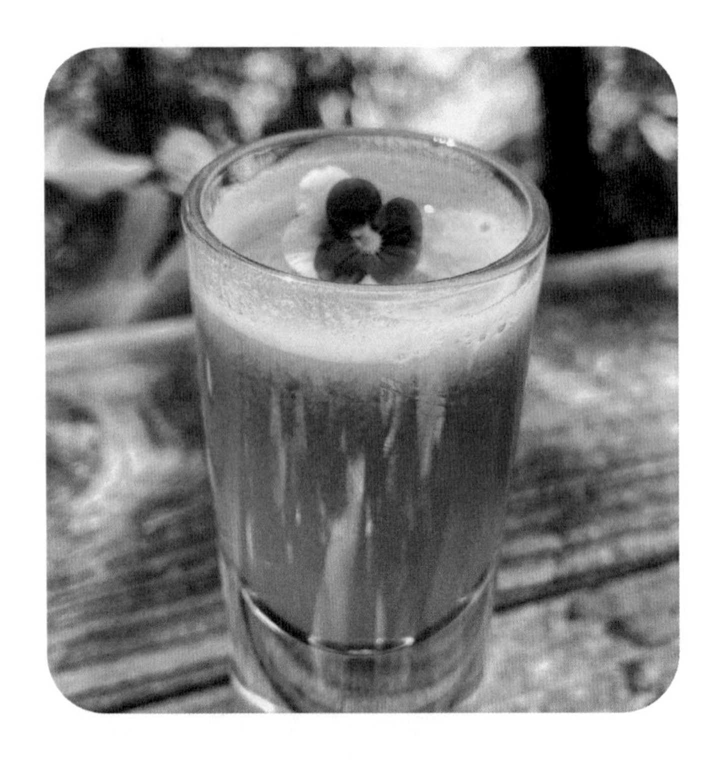

Zucchini Candy

A delicious and healthy snack. Zucchini and 100% juice are the only two ingredients.

Ingredients:

- large zucchini
- 100% juice (apple & purple grape are my favorite)

To Prepare:

Wash and dry zucchini. Remove seed pod and dice into half inch cubes. Place in pot and add 100% juice to cover all pieces. Add ½ C water. Bring to a low boil. Then turn heat down to simmer for 30-60 minutes.

Once translucent, drain and place mixture on dehydrator trays. (Or place in the sun to dry. Cover with a screen to keep bugs out.)

Set dehydrator to 130°F for 6-12 hours. Zucchini is done when it feels tacky, leathery, or dry to the touch.

For a spicy version, add cayenne pepper, cinnamon or ginger to the juice while simmering.

Store in a ziploc bag in the refrigerator.

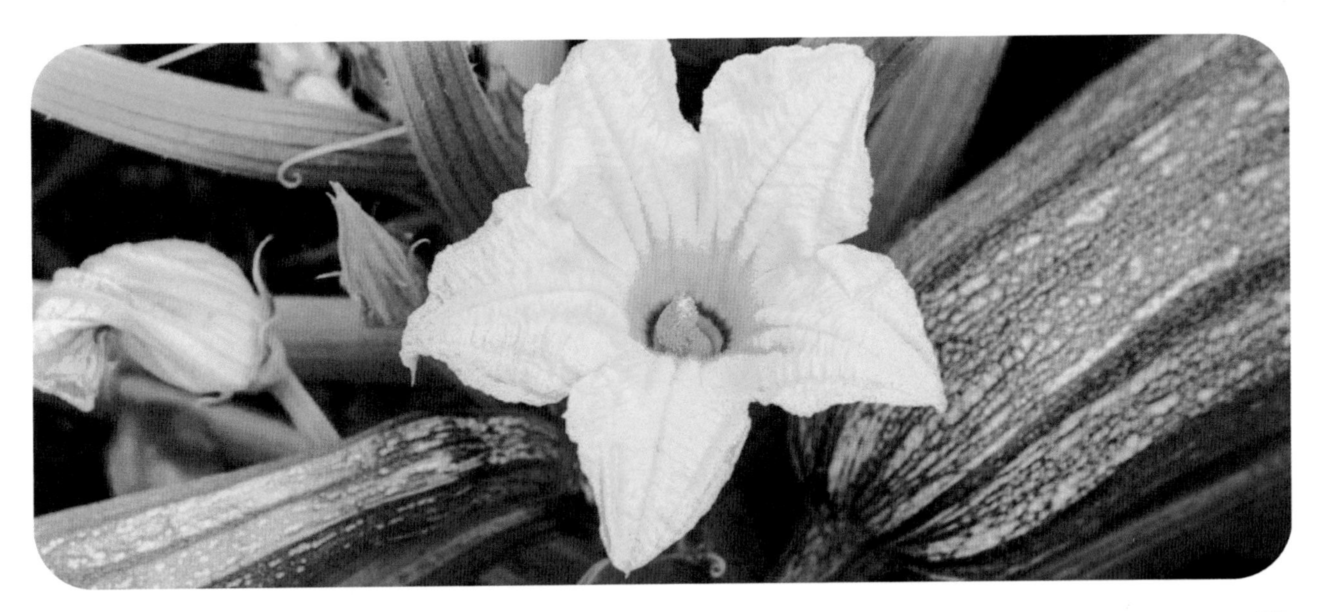

Dad's Easy Chicken Cacciatore

Monday night was the night my Dad was in the kitchen. This was one of his favorites.

Ingredients:

- 1 chicken, cut up
- salt, pepper
- flour
- 4 T olive oil
- 1 T butter
- 1 large onion
- 1 bell pepper
- 1 stalk of celery, finely chopped
- 1 garlic clove
- ¼ tsp sugar
- pinch of allspice or cinnamon
- ¼ C sherry or ½ C red wine
- 3 large tomatoes, peeled and cut
- season with rosemary, thyme and 1 bay leaf

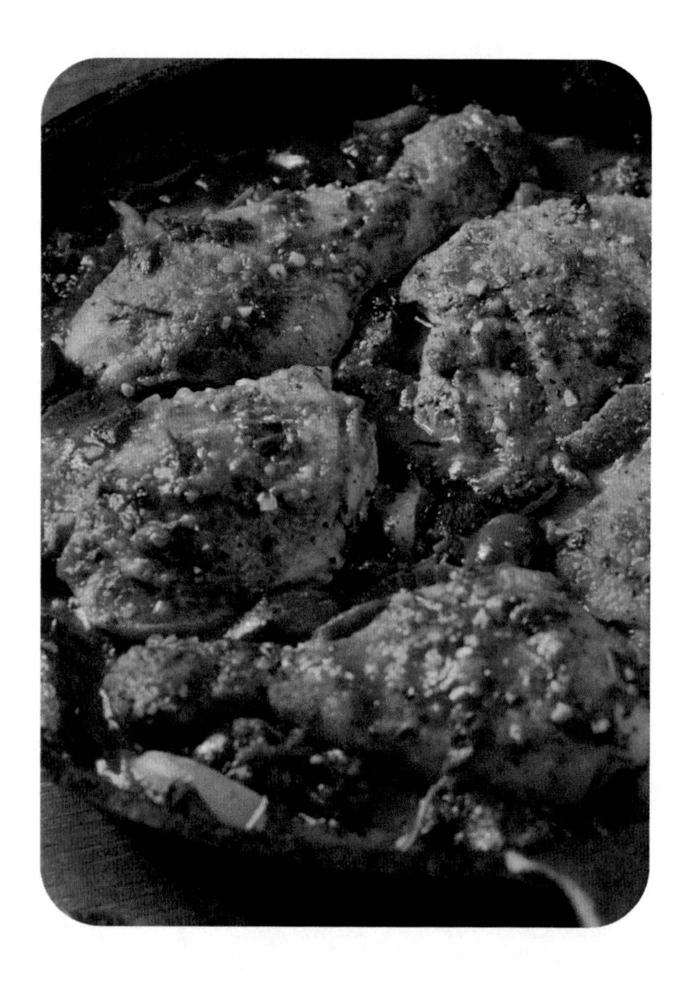

To Prepare:

Sprinkle chicken with salt, pepper and flour. Brown lightly in the olive oil & butter. Remove from pan and set aside.

To the pan add pepper, onion, celery and garlic. Sauté until onion is translucent. Add sugar, allspice/cinnamon, wine, chicken, tomatoes.

Cover and cook until chicken is tender—about 40-60 minutes, depending on size of pieces. If necessary, add more liquid (tomato juice, chicken broth or water) from time to time.

Season to taste. Serves 6.

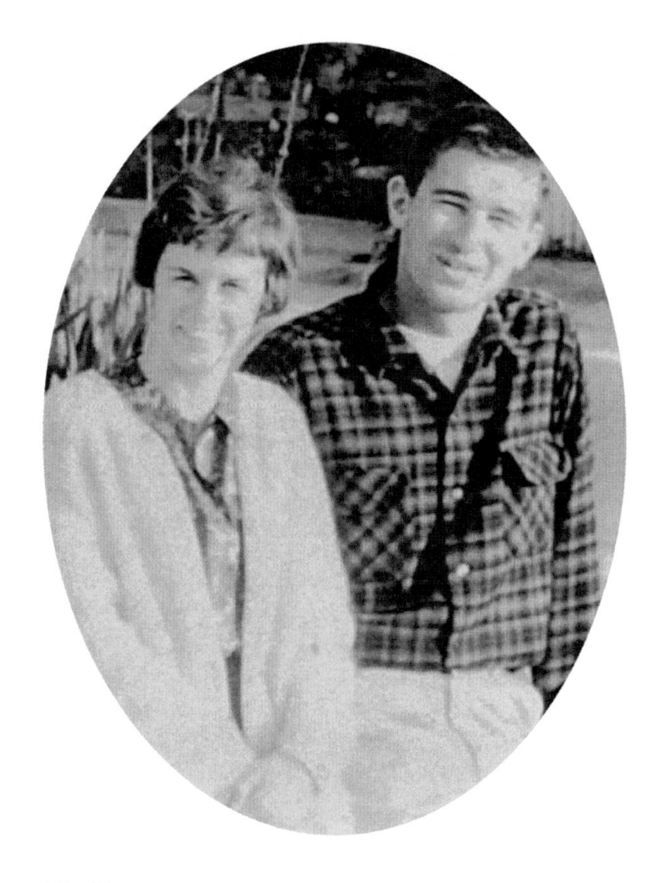

Mom's Gazpacho

Fresh from our garden . . .

Ingredients:

- 5 tomatoes
- 3 red bell peppers
- 3 cucumbers
- ½ red onion
- ¼ C olive oil
- oregano, cumin, chili powder to taste
- V-8 juice
- 1-2 jalapenos seeded, with some seeds if you like spicy
- **Optional**: (honey for a bit of sweetness depending on the tomatoes used).

To Prepare:

Mix in a food processor until desired consistency. Chill in a bowl for a minimum of 2 hours. Serve chilled and garnish with herbs, sour cream or avocado.

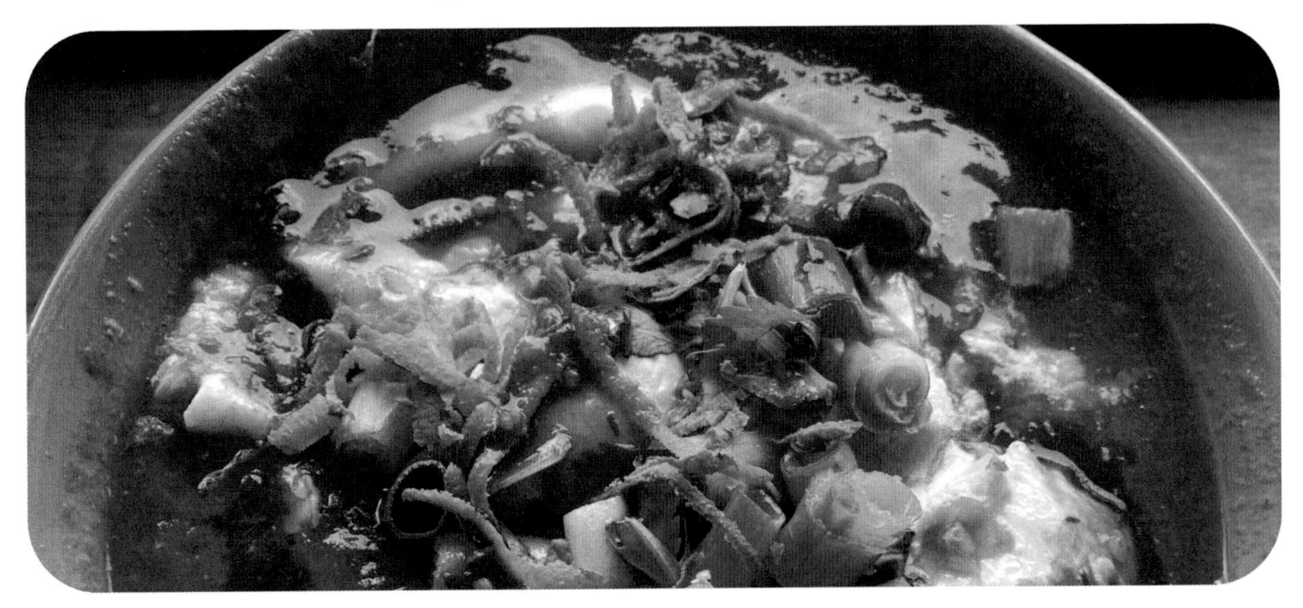

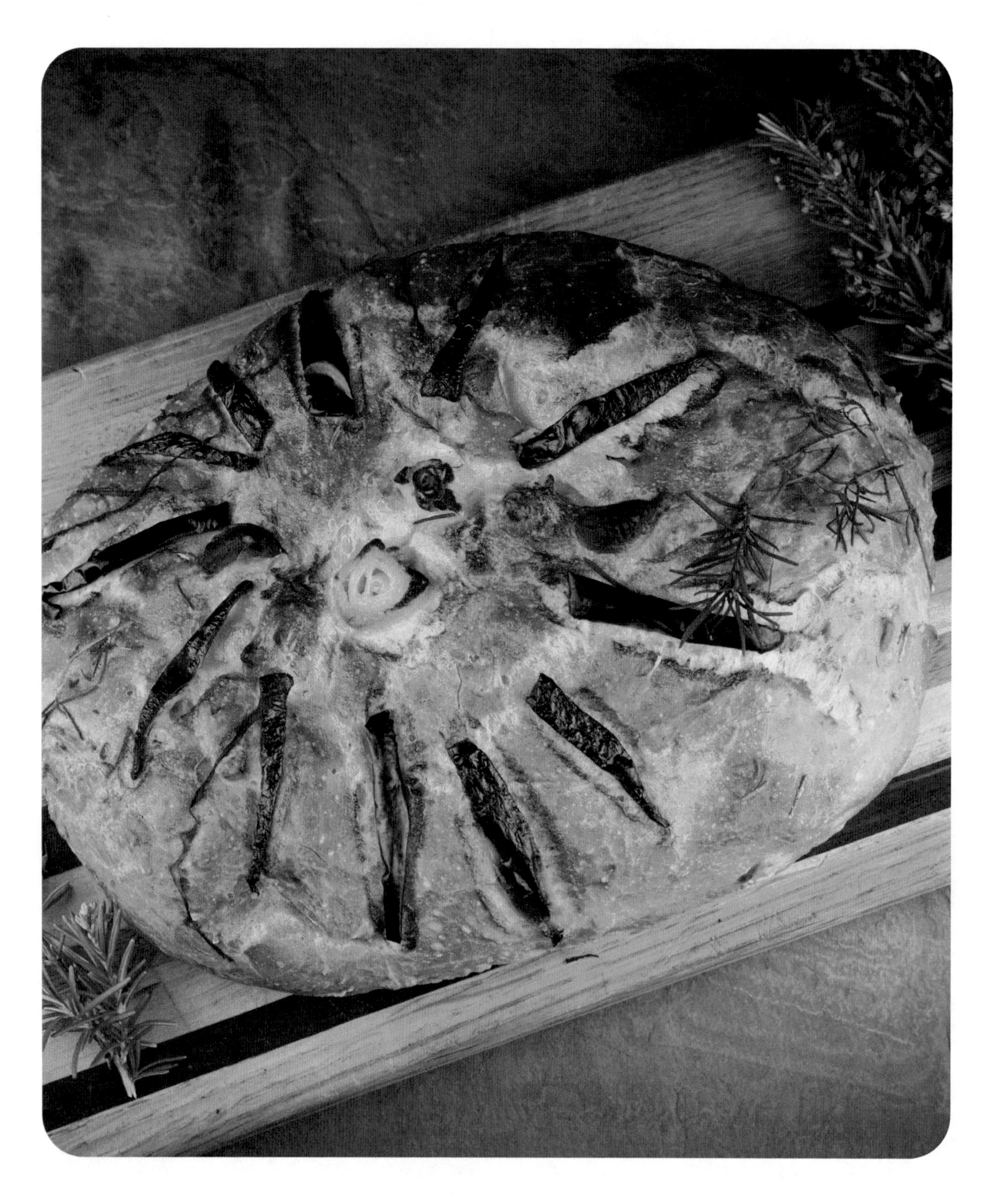

Artisan Bread

This bread is such a crowd-pleaser. Even the gluten-free have been known to splurge on these loaves. I always make an extra loaf and it disappears. Please use organic flour.

Ingredients:

- 3 C organic flour
- ¼ tsp active dry yeast
- 1 T organic sugar
- ½ tsp sea salt
- 1½ tsp garlic powder
- 1-2 C lukewarm water (test on hand)
- 1 T of your choice of herbs: scallion, rosemary, sage or thyme
- 1 small onion, thinly sliced in rounds
- garlic cloves

Supplies needed:

- 1 large mixing bowl
- 1 strong spatula for mixing
- Something to cover the bowl with while dough is rising
- Ceramic, glass, or cast-iron pan or baking pan with ovenproof lid

To Prepare:

Mix dry ingredients together. Add lukewarm water and mix with dry ingredients until you create a shaggy, sticky dough. Sprinkle in herbs. Cover bowl and let rise until double in size.

Preheat oven to 450°F. Place bread pan with lid in the oven and heat for 30 minutes.

Scrape the dough bowl and fold in the sides of the dough to create a round ball.

Remove hot pan from oven and pour in the bread dough. Using scissors, snip some lines in the top of the dough. Press in onion rounds, garlic cloves or a rosemary sprig into the top of the loaf. Do this step quickly or the bread will stick to pan! Preheating the pan allows for the loaf to be easily removed after the baking process is done. Place uncooked bread with lid into the oven and bake for 40 minutes. After 40 minutes remove the lid and bake for another 20 minutes until the crust is golden.

Remove from oven and let stand for at least 15 minutes before cutting into loaf. Serve with butter or vinaigrette dipping sauce.

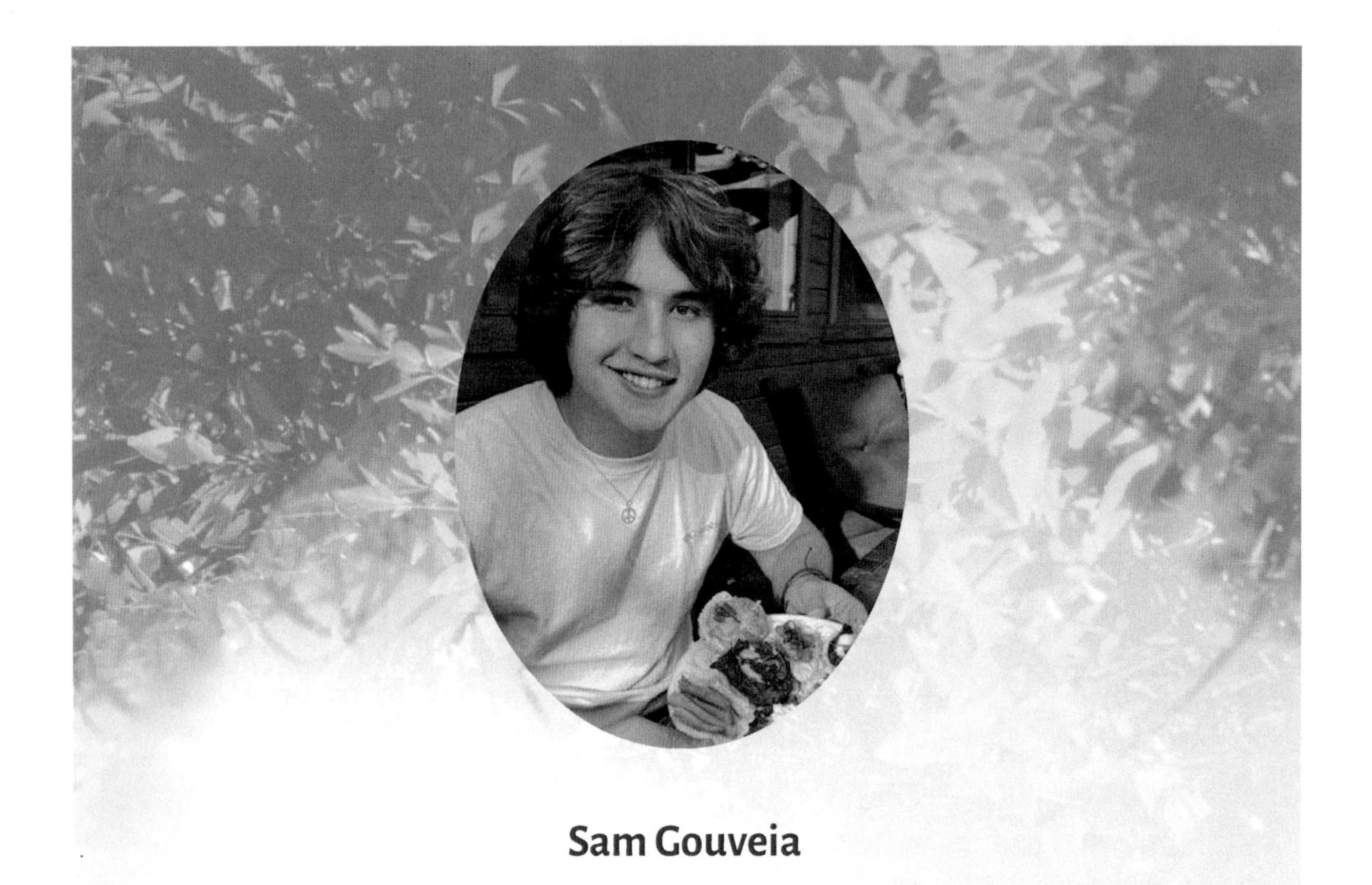

Sam Gouveia

Sam grew up on a farm in Grass Valley, California. He started foraging for greens when he started to walk! The first green he reached for—and stuffed into his mouth—was a grape leaf. His mom panicked and quickly went to the internet so see if her son had ingested anything toxic. What she found out was that, "grape leaves are very nutritious," and according to the USDA, "they are a great source of minerals such as calcium, iron and potassium. In addition, they are also high in fiber, folate and vitamins A and K. Grape leaves contain many phytochemicals and antioxidants that may contribute to overall positive health."

Since that day, Sam was hooked on picking greens, edible weeds and flowers. He would stack them up and create green wraps. When he started playing sports in high school, he became more curious about plant-based recipes for athletes and healthier versions of traditional recipes like pancakes, for example. The farm became a hub for Sam and his friends to learn about growing their own food, foraging the land, and cooking healthy dishes.

Sam is currently at Chico State pursuing a nutrition major. The following six recipes are his most often requested! Teen-approved. ☺

Lemon Banana & Blueberry Pancakes

Gluten-free & protein rich!

Ingredients:

- 1 C gluten-free pancake mix
  (we chose Pamela's brand made with almond meal)
- 1 large egg or 1 T flax seed
- ⅔ C water or nut/oat milk
- 1 T oil
- 1 medium banana, cut into thin rounds or diced
- blueberries
- 1 lemon, zested

To Prepare:

Mix flour, egg/flax seed, water/milk and oil together. Stir until all lumps are gone. Fold in bananas, blueberries and lemon zest. Batter should not be too thick or thin.

Pour onto oiled or buttered, heated pan. Butter creates a nice crispy edge. Look for the air bubbles that indicate it's time to flip the pancake. Top with jam or real maple syrup.

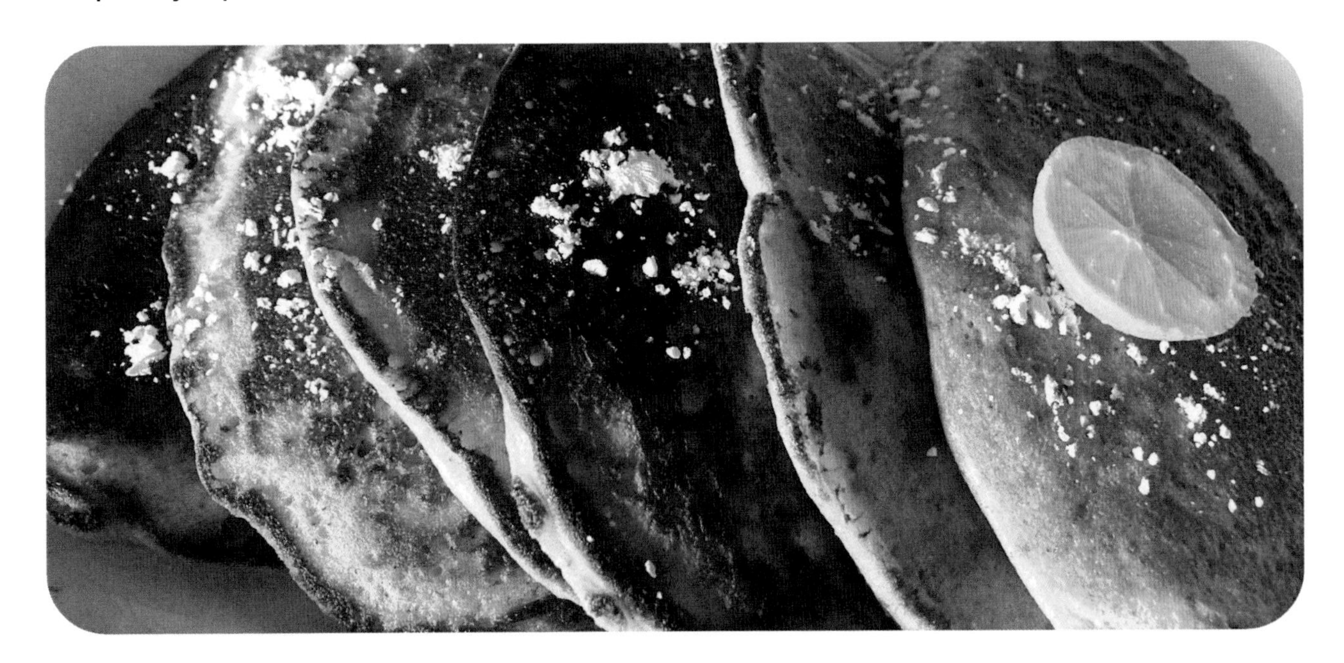

Coconut & Seed Breakfast Bars

Plant-based & gluten-free!

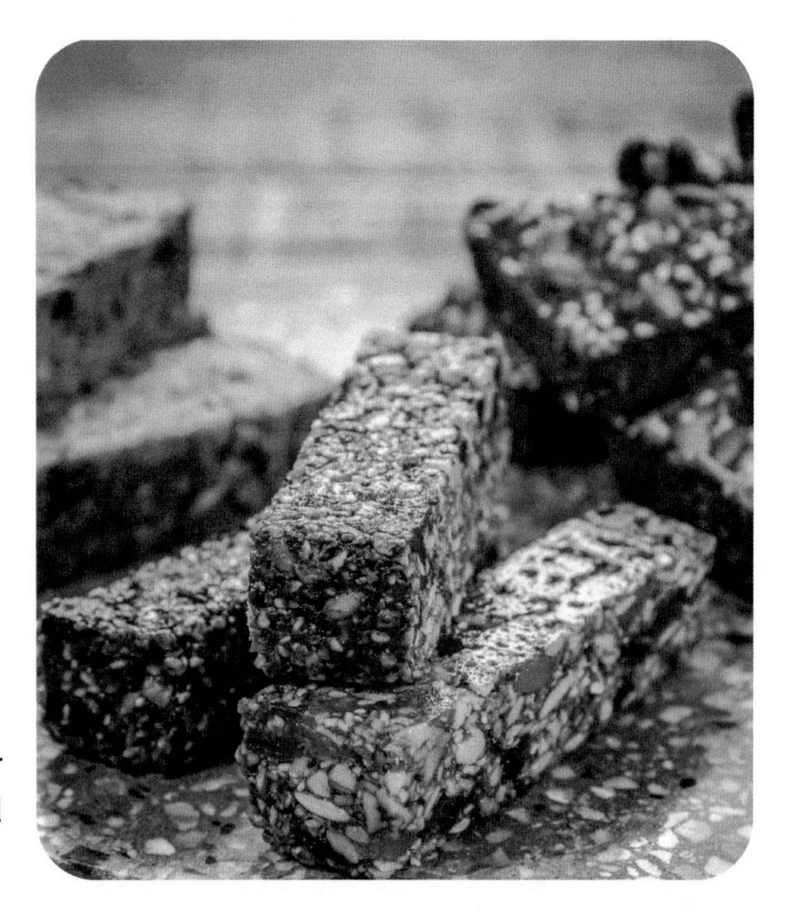

Ingredients:

- 2 C shredded coconut
- ½ C sunflower seeds
- ¼ C sesame seeds
- 2 T coconut oil
- ¼ C arrowroot starch or chickpea flour
- ¼ C honey or maple syrup
- ½ tsp vanilla
- ½ tsp lemon zest
- pinch of sea salt

To Prepare:

Mix coconut in food processor until it becomes clumpy and starts to stick together.

Add the rest of the ingredients and pulse to blend.

Scoop into rounds and place on a cookie sheet lined with parchment paper.

Bake at 350°F for 10-15 minutes or until golden brown.

Let cool and serve at room temperature.

Baked Potato with Avocado

Ingredients:

- large, organic Russett potatoes
- avocado, mashed
- green onions, sliced
- lemon zest
- salt, pepper and garlic powder

To Prepare:

Pierce potatoes with fork and rub with olive oil, salt, pepper, rosemary/herbs and garlic powder.

Bake at 425°F for 1 hour or until tender.

Slice the top open and fill with mashed avocado, sliced green onion, lemon zest, salt, pepper, and garlic powder.

Optional: squeeze with fresh lemon juice for a moister potato.

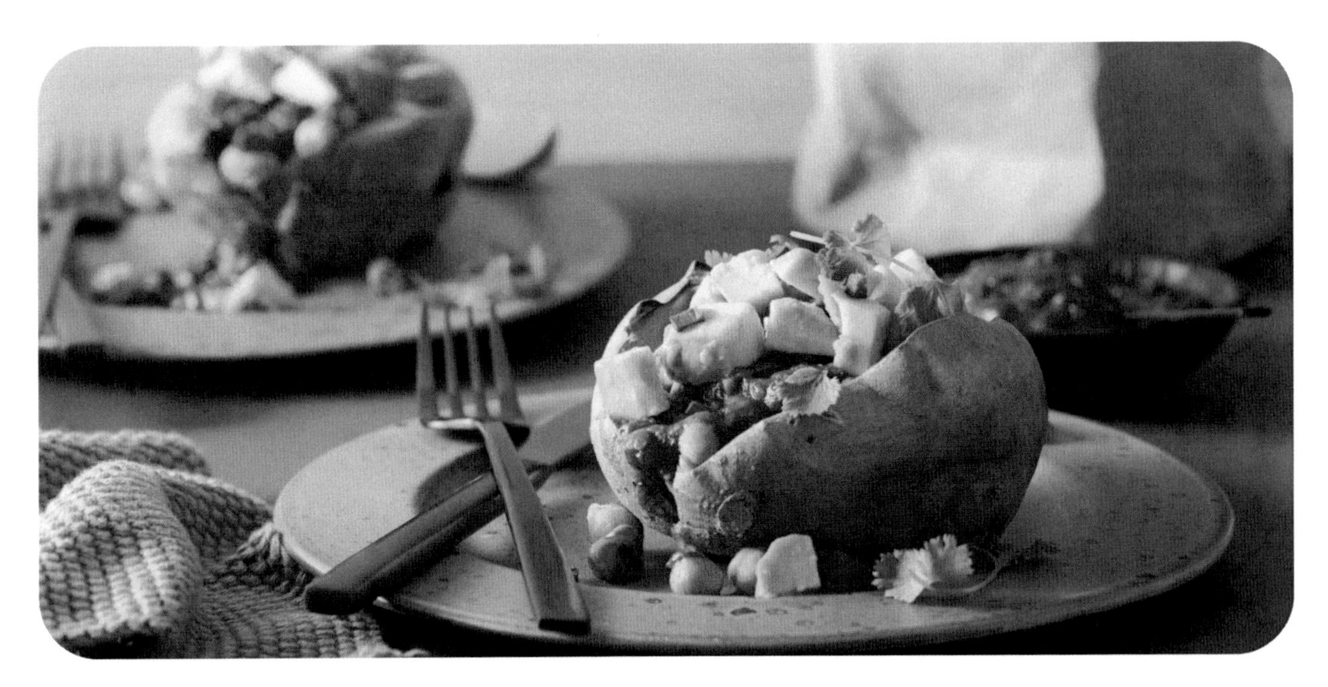

Chickpea Salad Sandwich

Plant-based!

Ingredients:

- 2 T tahini
- 1 tsp Dijon mustard
- 1 garlic clove
- 1 T capers
- 1 green onion
- 2 T of cilantro or parsley
- 2 T lemon juice + lemon zest
- salt & pepper, to taste

To Prepare:

Pulse all ingredients in a food processor until desired consistency. We like ours to be a bit chunky. Wrap in a tortilla, lettuce leaf, or spread on bread.

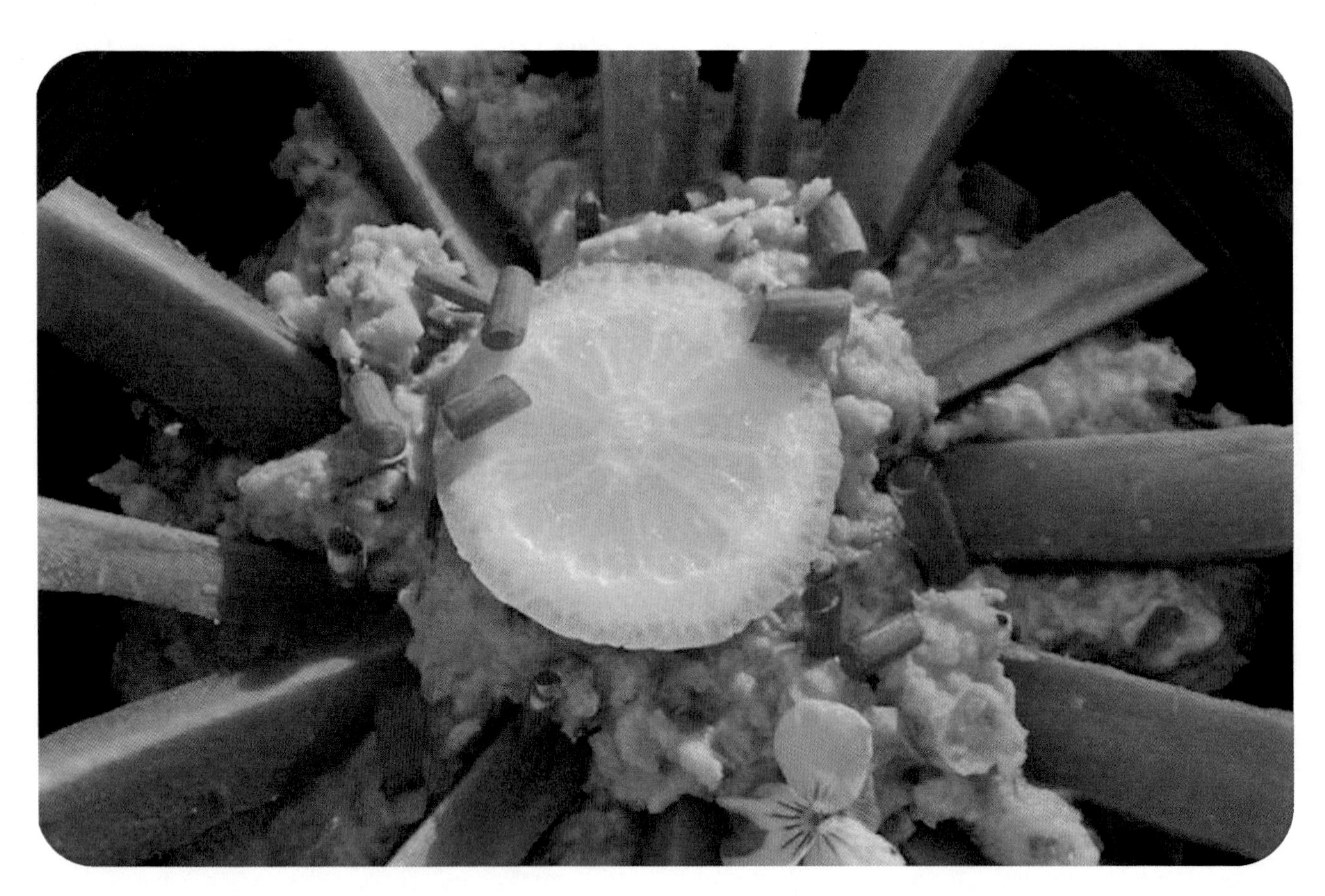

Cabbage Burgers

Plant-based & gluten-free!

Ingredients:

- 4 C purple cabbage, chopped
- 2 eggs
- 1 medium onion (yellow, white or purple), diced
- 1 garlic clove, diced
- ⅓ C chickpea/ garbanzo flour
- ½ tsp each: black pepper, salt, paprika, cumin, garlic powder

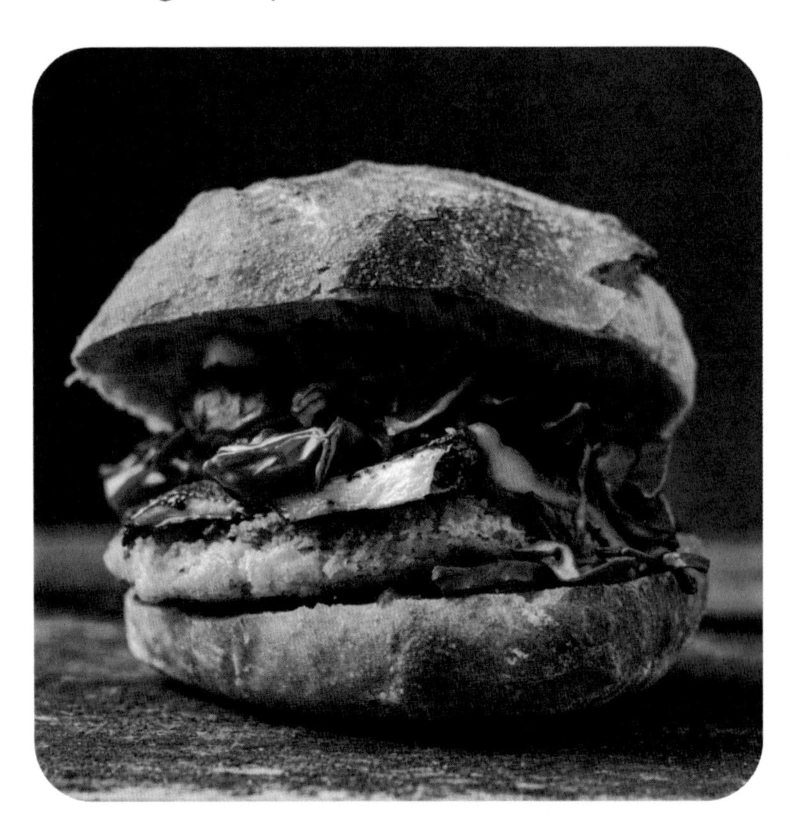

To Prepare:

Steam cabbage for 10 minutes or until soft and tender. Remove and put into a bowl to cool slightly.

Meanwhile, chop onion and sauté in a frying pan until soft and translucent. Add diced garlic and cook for another 2 minutes.

When cabbage is cool you may need to squeeze the excess water out of it, so it forms into patties.

Combine all of the ingredients together and mix well. Shape into balls or patties.

Heat a pan with coconut oil and fry on low to medium heat until golden on both sides. Use as burgers, sliders, or meat balls. Enjoy!

Crazy Delicious Healthy Bowls!

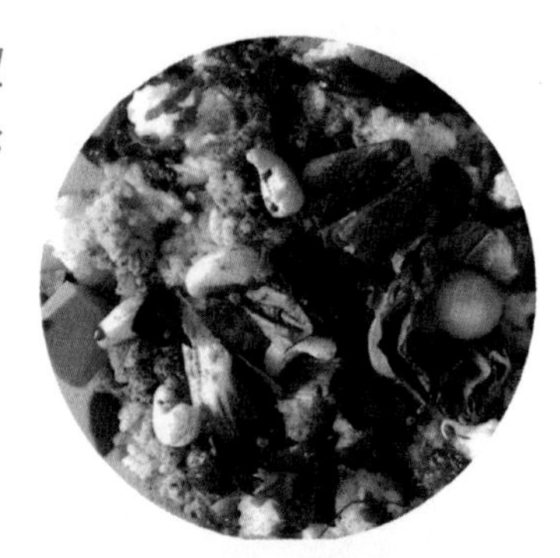

These rice bowls are a fun way to combine healthy, colorful ingredients that you have on hand. Different sauces (recipes are in this book) can be made and frozen ahead of time for a variety of themed bowls during the week. Using riced cauliflower, or brown or white rice, create a "canvas" to decorate with your favorite toppings.

Ingredients:

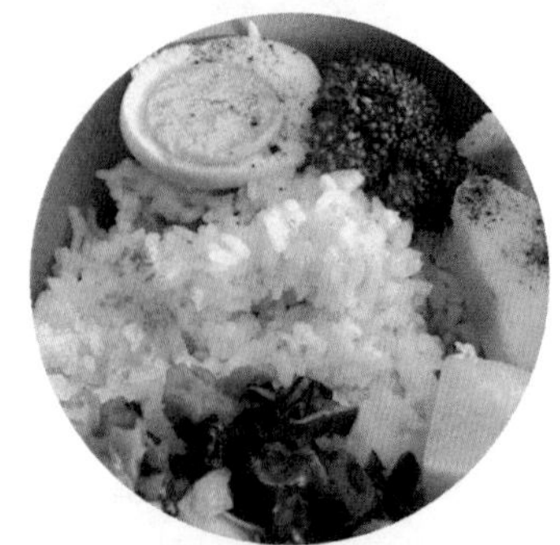

Try incorporating these six categories for Fiesta, Buddha, Italian, Thai and Vegan themed bowls.

1. **Protein:** meat, chicken, fish, egg or plant-based protein like tofu, tempeh, black beans or pinto beans

2. **Raw or steamed veggies:** broccoli, sweet potato, potato, radish, carrots, squash, turnips, red and green cabbage, spinach, kale, cucumber, celery, beets and peas

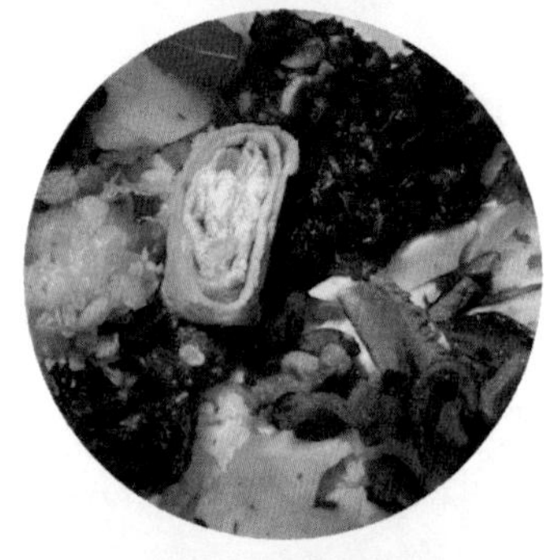

3. **Fruit:** pineapple, pickled watermelon, mango, citrus or apple

4. **Ferments:** sauerkraut, kimchi, pickled beets, ginger and veggies

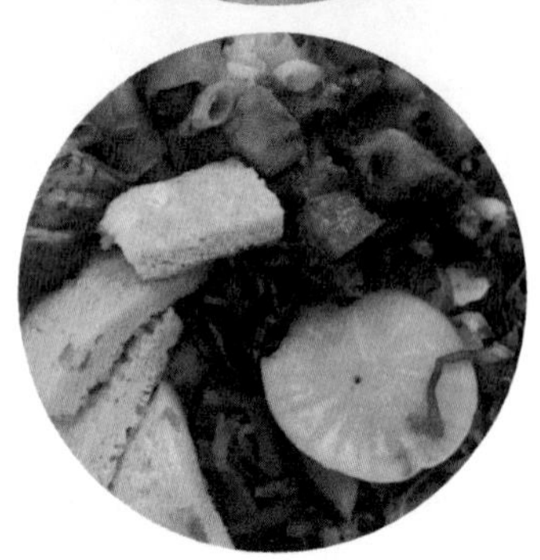

5. **Nutrient-dense herbs & spices:** cilantro, parsley, green onion, mint, turmeric, paprika, or cayenne pepper

6. Drizzle with a **themed sauce** for international bowls: Thai peanut, chimichurri, creamy salsa, cashew "cheese", avocado ranch, or dressing of your choice.

Sam's Favorite Edible Flowers

For garnishing & for health!

These flowers can be dried, candied, pressed and used for cocktails, desserts and salads:

- Viola
- Pansy
- Calendula
- Mustard
- Borage
- Nasturtium
- Marigold
- Arugula
- Bachelor Buttons
- Roses
- Pineapple Guava

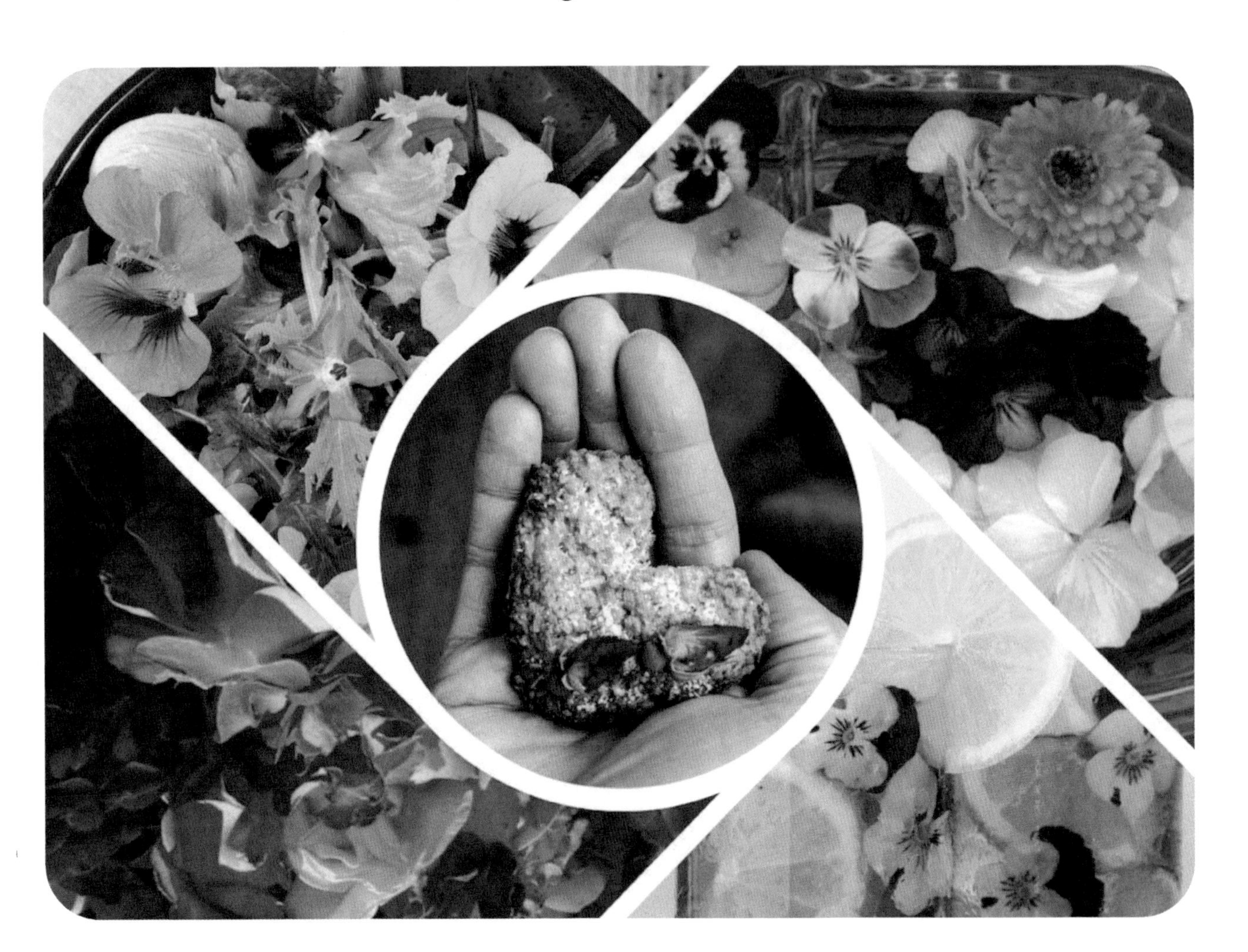

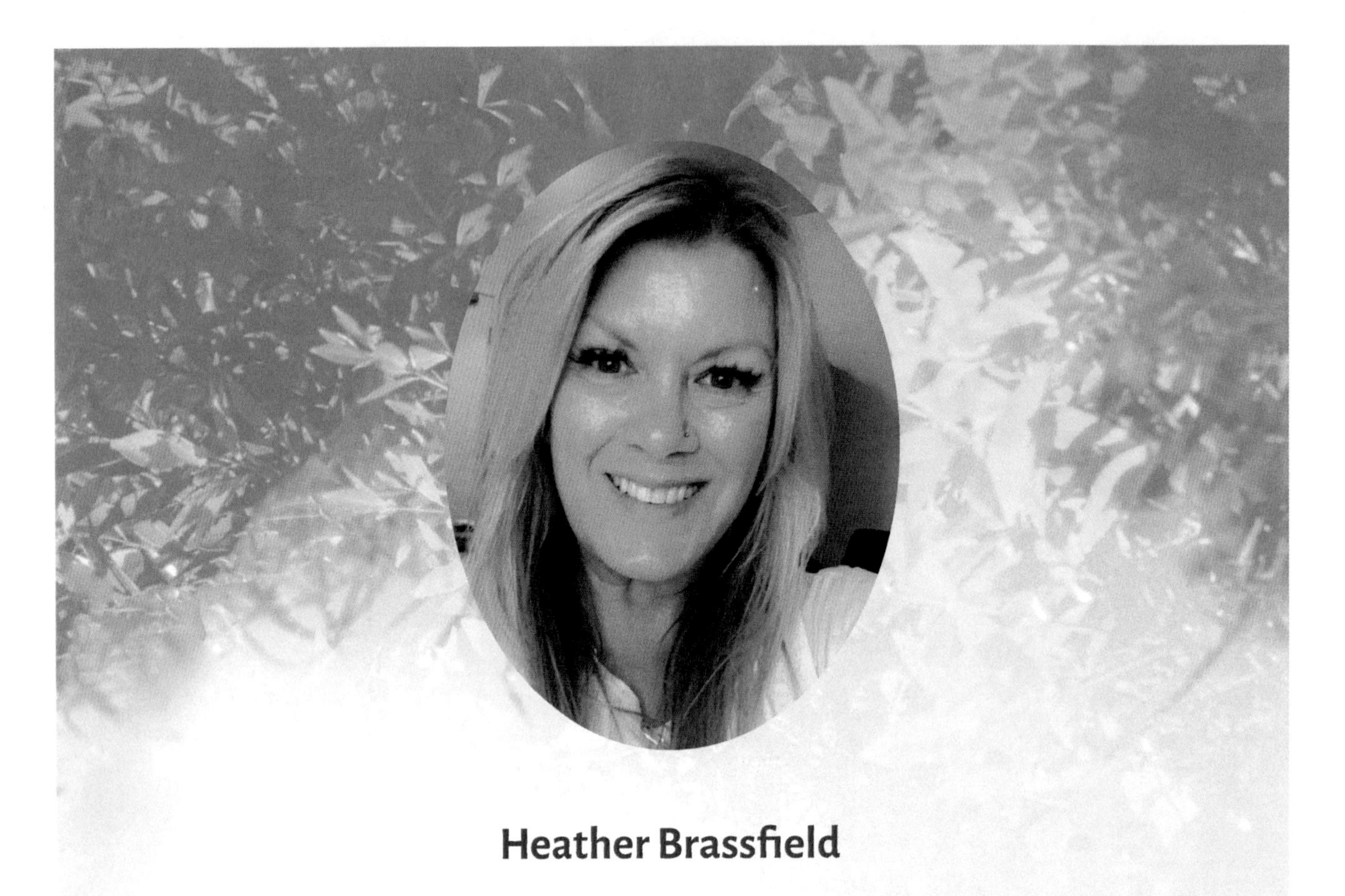

Heather Brassfield

In 2014, I purchased a house here in Nevada City, CA and made it into a small farm and Airbnb. I knew I wanted to move here one day, when I came to visit a friend when I was 16.

I started getting into nutrition in 2005. I was feeling ill; my face was puffy and I was tired all the time. I worked at a chiropractic office and had been learning about new ways of healing and eating and I knew that was the way to go for me. I found out about a wonderful holistic doctor who ended up diagnosing me with candida. I followed her protocol and it worked. I was better within a couple of weeks. This started my dive into nutrition, and not the USDA kind of nutrition. Since then, I have been following a plant-based diet and even 80% raw. I feel so amazing on a whole plant-food-based diet. I have a very busy life and travel, so I am not perfect on this way of life, but I do my best.

I have submitted a few raw vegan sauce recipes to this cookbook for people who want to have amazing non-dairy sauces on their plant-based meals. These sauces are what have kept me on track, and they are good on everything, hot or cold. They are satisfying and super yummy and I hope you like them too.

Instagram: Brassflower_farm

Raw Sour Cream

You can replace the cashews with PB2 Powdered Cashew Butter. Make the paste into the same amount as the recipe calls for. It's a fraction of the fat and calories and tastes great. You can get it on Amazon.

Ingredients:

- ½ C raw cashews, soaked overnight
- 1 small clove garlic
- 1 tsp apple cider vinegar or ½ tsp lemon juiced
- pinch salt
- ¼ C unsweetened plant milk

To Prepare:

Blend until creamy. To make Alfredo, just add more garlic and pour over raw kelp noodles for a delicious meal.

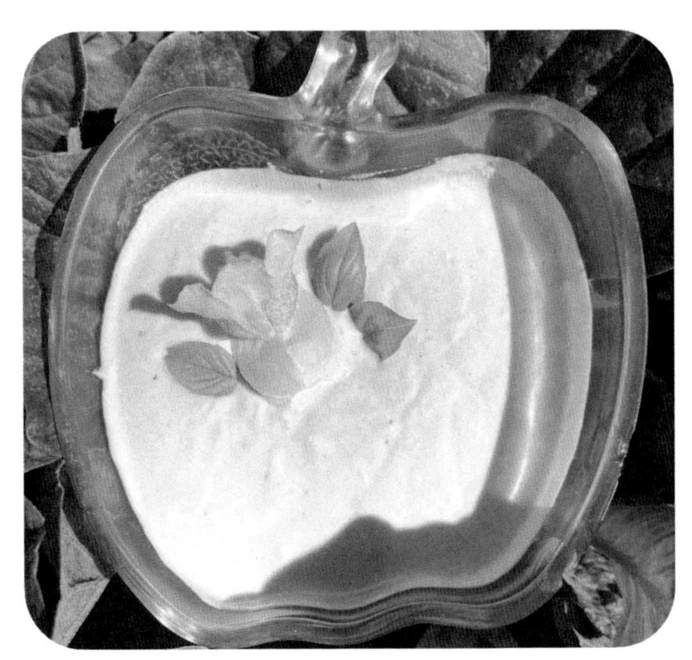

Raw Vegan Ranch Dressing

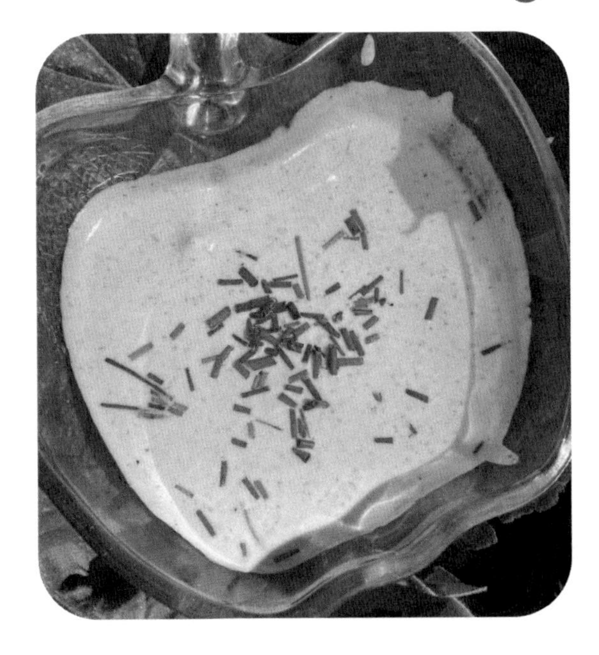

Ingredients:

Use the sour cream recipe. Add:

- ¼ tsp basil
- ¼ tsp chives
- ¼ tsp dill
- 1 clove garlic
- ⅛ C water, or more depending on desired consistency

To Prepare:

Blend until creamy. Add more chives and/or dill and stir in.

Yummy Raw Almond Dressing

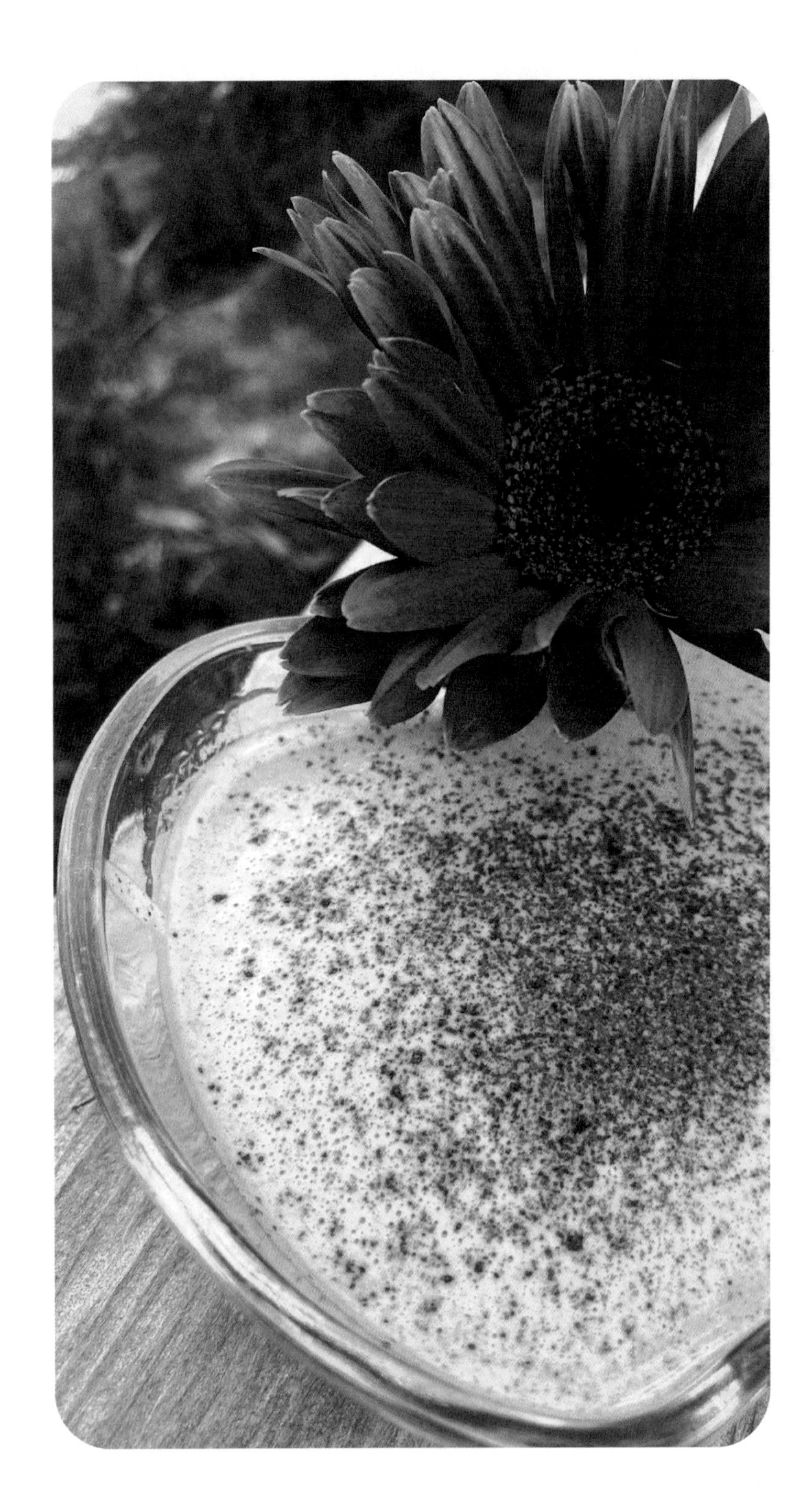

Ingredients:

- ½ C raw almond butter (not roasted). You can also use raw tahini.
- ½ C water
- 1 tsp apple cider vinegar
- 2 tsp nama shoyu (soy sauce)
- ¼ C lemon juice
- 2 cloves garlic
- **Optional**: for a sweeter dressing add ½ T coconut aminos or maple syrup.

To Prepare:

Blend into a dressing.

Add cayenne to taste, if desired.

The Best Vegan Cheese Sauce

This is such an amazing sauce. Add to macaroni for mac 'n cheese, or to top your tacos, wrap, or veggie sushi. If you want to make this lower fat you can use PB2 Cashew Powder. It works great, and has a fraction of the fat and calories, but it is not raw.

Ingredients:

- ½ C raw soaked cashews
- ¼ C jarred roasted bell pepper (you can use raw to stay raw)
- ½ tsp onion powder
- 4 T nutritional yeast
- 1 clove garlic
- ½ lemon, juiced
- ¼ C unsweetened plant milk

To Prepare: Blend until smooth.

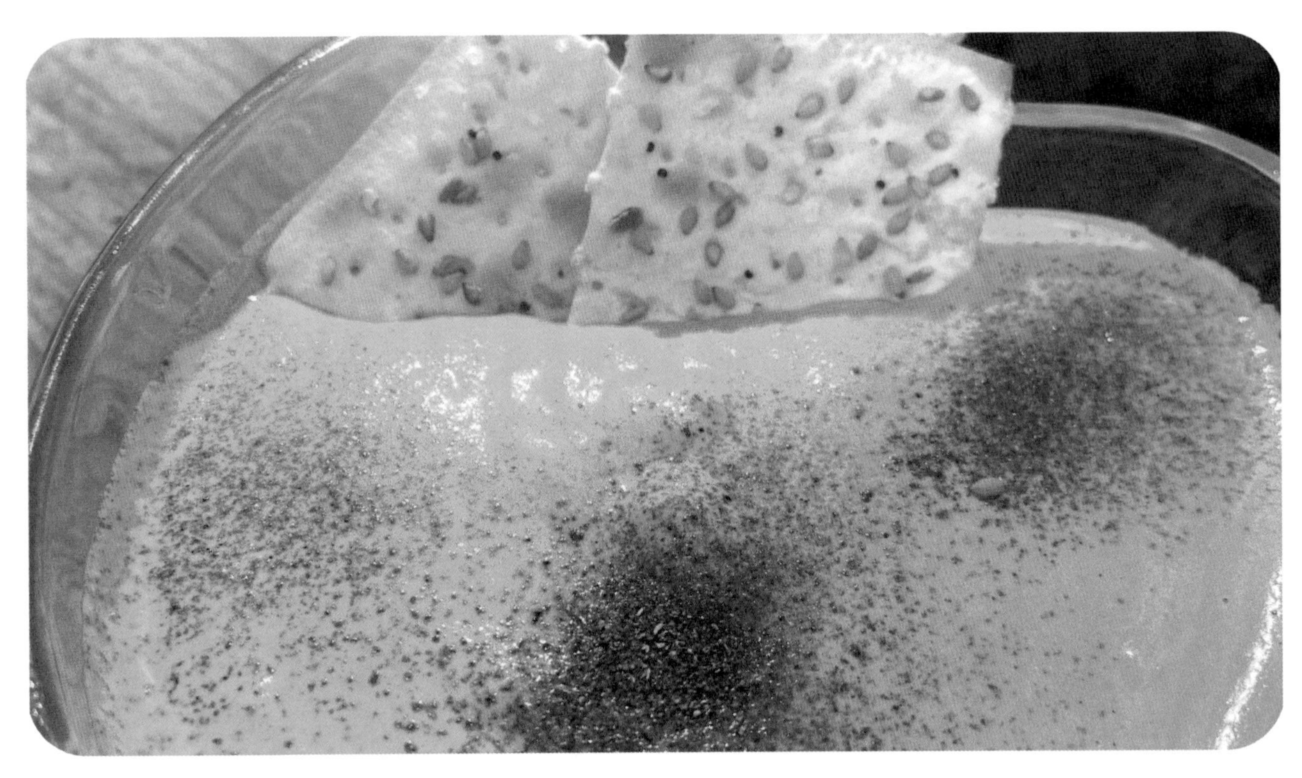

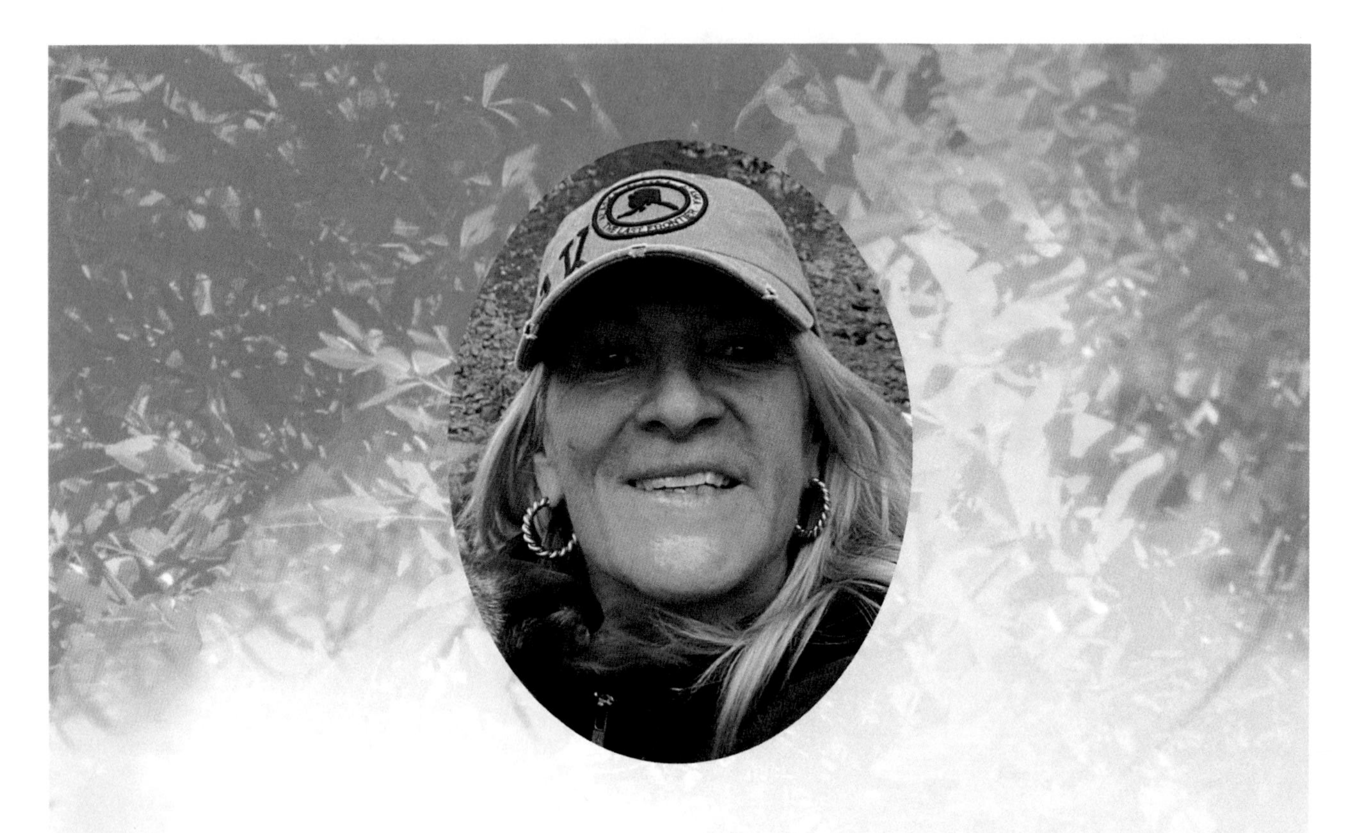

Linda Nelson-Bracken

Linda Nelson-Bracken is a multi-lingual (English, Italian, Spanish) entrepreneur and international real estate investor. Multiple project locations include California, Alaska, several Italian cities, and recently, Costa Rica. She specializes in creatively transforming and remodeling using upcycling to improve real estate value.

Linda is currently a Super Host and manages several Airbnb listings. She also hosts retreats, and coordinates events which include real estate strategies, wellness, and Christian belief.

4

The Health Benefits of Living in a Blue Zone

Linda Nelson-Bracken

"But the Holy Spirit produces this kind of Fruits in our lives:
Love, Peace, Joy , Patience, Kindness Goodness, Faithfulness, Gentleness, and Self Control."

~ Galatians 5:22

I have lived an incredible, colorful life and for as long as I can remember, the Holy Spirit has led me and used me through creativity and entrepreneurial ideas. Thanks to our parents, Susan (Gouveia) and I had access to a multitude of supplies, which afforded us a blank canvas for endless possibilities, forming who we are today: creative, confident, female entrepreneurs.

With easels, paints, a garden, building supplies, a chicken coop and more, our home in Danville, California was the playground for our entrepreneurial endeavors. At the age of 13, my older sister, Susan, had this cool summer crafts class. I got to hang out, help, and witness how people gave her money to have fun! Most importantly, she touched our community and encouraged future artists. I loved watching her count the money in the jar at the end of the summer.

Having no interest in institutionalized schooling, and a yearning to learn to cook and design, the Holy Spirit directed me to Italy at age 20. It was there I met Vanni, my handsome "Italian Souvenir," (as he was referred to). He was a cross between Bruce Willis and John Travolta. I lived with his family and learned Italian by cooking and sewing.

Working my way into a position as a dynamite Murano glass sales agent, I was inspired by the beauty of the glass and began designing jewelry and exporting it internationally. When the currency exchange rate made this no longer advantageous, the Holy Spirit led me to teach. When I learned I did not have the necessary credentials, I opened my own school. My students ranged from 3-80 years old. We took the youth on trips to London, introducing them to culture, hands-on.

When I was invited to the local middle school to teach in Venice Italy, my heart grew a thousand sizes. I had no idea how to do this, but the Holy Spirit led me. Then, sitting on the beach one day, I overheard a conversation that the 5-star hotel Cipriani needed a kids' activity program. My summers, many years ago helping my sister, gave me the courage to write a killer business plan, and I landed a gig where my 5-year-old son worked with me, and hung out with VIP families while I taught crafts and cooking. Massimo was becoming accustomed to this level of hospitality and this was his foundation and standard. I was then sent to the sister hotels located in Portofino, Florence, Ravenna and Sicily to open my program, and enjoy the 5-star locations. It was beyond amazing! But something was missing: working with rich people was not feeling fulfilling for me. I wanted to work with the disadvantaged.

During this entire journey I purchased real estate, remodeled and flipped property, on an average of every three years. The Holy Spirit told me when to buy and when to sell. Places such as Venice, California and, most recently Costa Rica, have been on my investment radar. For years I dreamed of raising my kids in a Spanish-speaking country and considered moving to Spain.

When Vanni and I could no longer make our marriage work, I painfully returned to California, to be around family. But my heart's desire was to incorporate Spanish. Starting anew was difficult, leaving my youngest, Massimo, behind and fleeing with my oldest, Matteo. I did what I knew: I bought a multi-unit rental property . . . in Grass Valley.

Somewhere along the way, Matteo excitedly called me from Costa Rica, "Ma, you gotta buy a place here in Montezuma or Santa Teresa!" Next thing I knew I was standing in the TSA line in Costa Rica talking with a group of teenagers wearing matching shirts. They were so happy, and confident. They were on a mission trip to teach local kids crafts, love on them, and spread the word of Jesus. All of it sounded amazing . . . but who was this Jesus guy?

I wanted a retreat property where I could host youth and we could teach local kids English and cooking. The realtor took me to one property located exactly between Santa Teresa and Montezuma—a retreat property that had been on the market for three years. That was it!

After a chaotic chapter in my life, I sold my beautiful, lucrative investment in

Grass Valley and downsized to my black convertible BMW and drove to Vegas. On the drive, the Holy Spirit told me, "Live with families and just serve them. Observe how they "Eat, Love and Pray." At this point, my two sons were estranged from me, I had lost $300,000 to my ex-boyfriend, and I needed to get away from our toxic relationship. What did I have to lose?

Upon arrival in Vegas, I received an email from a woman I didn't know very well—my current "boyfriend's" sister. She was visiting LA for a conference. I saw this divine appointment as an opportunity for me to ask for help, and untangle myself from her brother's manipulative spirit. Driving down the Pacific Coast Highway together, I declined the invitation to stay with her in Alaska and receive council and coaching. (I thought to myself, *who even lives in Alaska?!*) Minutes later, my "check engine" light popped on, and I was at a Malibu mechanic, learning my car would need to be there for 10 days, while they sorted out the problem. Malibu . . . *yuck, who even lives in Malibu!?* I thought.

Next thing I knew, I was on a plane to Alaska. My friend reported that her older brother had just suffered a heart attack. I knew that this was my first assignment for me to serve. It was there, in Alaska, that I felt the presence of God. I couldn't explain it. I could hear him; I could feel him. Living with my (ex) boyfriend's family introduced me to reading the Bible and becoming curious about a relationship with God—the spiritual father I never really knew, but felt, who guided me, when I listened. I cooked, dog-sat, taught the children to knit, and served when there were church guest speakers . . . and I gave my heart to Jesus.

Going to church, praying, and reading the Bible RADICALLY changed my life.

Within a month Massimo and Matteo were back in my life. I purchased a beautiful cabin property on a lake and Massimo came to live with me. In this large single room, with an outhouse and wood-burning stove for warmth, we did COVID. We made a living by buying storage units and selling the contents on Market Place. Massimo had talent and we were having fun.

As the snow started to fall, my water pipes froze, and more and more wood needed to be split. I realized I had NO business living in these circumstances alone with my 16-year-old. I desired a help mate: a husband, a person to manage my projects. I spent most of my days in Home Depot, so I was hopeful to meet a handyman or construction worker. In Alaska there are 10 men to every woman. The odds made sense. Then I learned a key Alaskan saying, "The odds are good, but the goods are odd!"

Back to church and back to prayer I went. I took a prayer request and wrote down very specific requirements for the man I wanted. I put it in the bucket and walked up to say hello to the pastor, since I hadn't been in church for a while. He blurted out, "Are you dating anyone? You should stalk my brother Chris on Instagram. He lives in Malibu, and works as a manager for some crazy Venetian guys." That was all the information I needed. The details I would work out. We Facetime-dated for three weeks. Drinking coffee on my beautiful lakeside terrace, the Holy Spirit told me to go get my BMW in California and drive to Malibu to check this dude out. I texted him, with no response.

So, back on the plane I went. Chris and I met, and we felt like old friends who had known each other for years. Within two months, he moved to Alaska, and I was soon married to my awesome husband, Chris, from Malibu, who shares the same love for hospitality, real estate, cooking, and serving God. We currently spend our life running a lakefront summer cabin business in Alaska and an Airbnb in Costa Rica. We are Kingdom Hospitality, offering retreats that incorporate education of real estate, fitness, food, finance, and vision with a heart of serving.

PURA VIDA! RECIPES

One of the most important reasons I chose to live in Costa Rica is because it is a Blue Zone. Meaning, the Nicoya Peninsula enjoys a balance of Family, Fitness, Food and Faith, making these "ingredients" the secret to health and longevity. Also, many of my favorite foods thrive here: avocados, mangos, ginger, turmeric, pineapples, bananas, cabbage, papaya, plantains, hibiscus, cilantro, and many more live in my garden! I don't grow them, they live here. My recipes include mainly these ingredients and offer great combinations for leftovers and new creations the next day.

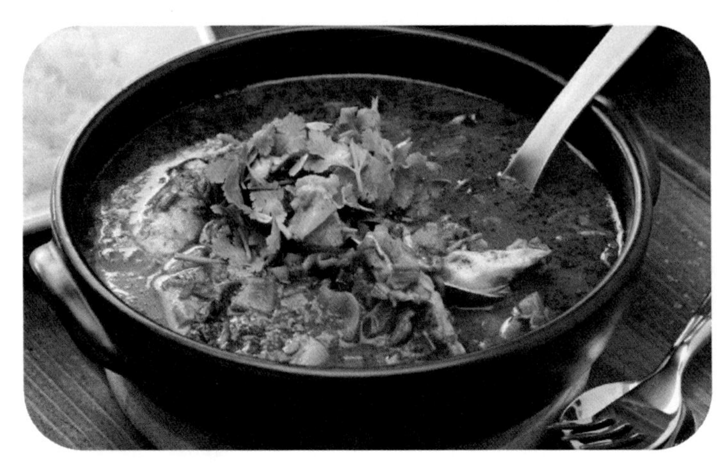

Fish Stew

This fish stew recipe follows me everywhere! From my years living in Venice, Italy and enjoying all the fresh fish; to Alaska with cod and salmon; to Costa Rica with tuna and dorado. I love recipes that are quick and tasty and incorporate the local catch of the day.

Ingredients:

- 1 lb. fish filets
- 1 C each, finely diced: onion, carrot, celery, potato, canned tomatoes
- 2 T olive oil
- garlic, oregano, basil, cayenne pepper, salt and pepper as palate desires

To Prepare:

In a large pot, sauté veggies, 1 fish filet, and spices in olive oil until veggies are soft (about 10 minutes). Stir and break up the filet so it flavors the stock.

Add water to preference (sometimes I prefer the stew thick, as a main course, and sometimes more liquid). Allow to simmer 30 minutes. Add remaining cubed filets and simmer an additional 15 minutes.

Serve with hot crusty bread, or warm tortillas. Great the next day!

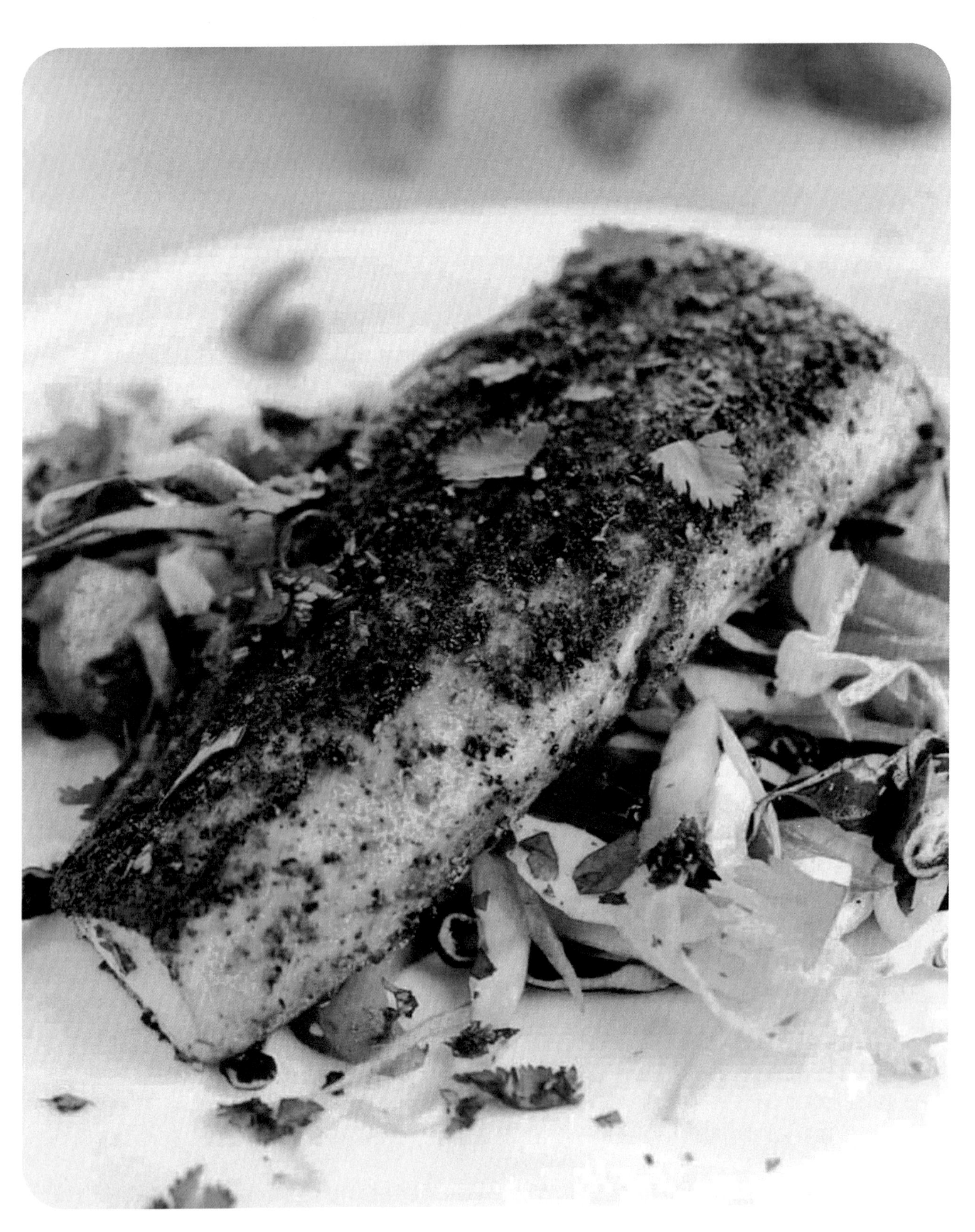

Seared Dorado

This recipe is perfect for using the catch of the day: sailfish, blue marlin, tuna, dorado or shrimp. We cook plenty of fish for leftovers used in fish tacos, cold salads or spreads. Serve with coleslaw.

Ingredients:

- 1 tsp smoked paprika
- 1 tsp dried thyme
- ½ tsp garlic powder
- ½ tsp freshly ground pepper
- ½ tsp salt
- ¼ tsp cayenne
- ¼ tsp chili
- 4-6 snapper fillets, or fish of choice (more for leftovers)
- avocado slices for garnish
- coconut oil for greasing pan

Coleslaw Ingredients:

- 2 C each green and purple cabbage, shredded
- 2 T apple cider vinegar
- ginger, to taste, shredded
- 1 T honey
- ½ T Dijon mustard
- ½ tsp ground pepper (I like lots!)
- ¼ C mayonnaise
- salt, pepper
- ½ C pineapple, mango or papaya, finely chopped
- 1 red bell pepper, diced
- 1 carrot, shredded

To Prepare:

Preheat broiler. Coat a rimmed baking sheet with coconut oil. In a small bowl combine spices and rub the mixture on fish filets.

Shred cabbage into a large bowl, add salt and pepper. Massage mixture for 3 minutes. This tenderizes and softens the cabbage. Stir in mayonnaise, mustard, vinegar, honey, fruit and red pepper.

Preheat oven to 400°F and bake fish for 10 minutes.

Serve with coleslaw. Take it another step and serve it with heated corn or flour tortillas and salsa, for a bomb fish taco!

Quinoa Rice & Couscous Salad

Ingredients:

- ½ C each: cooked quinoa, rice and couscous
- ¼ C each: chopped tomatoes, red onion, carrots, celery, beans
- ¼ C chopped parsley and basil combined
- 2-3 T olive oil
- salt and pepper to taste

To Prepare:

Cook rice, quinoa, and couscous separately according to directions.

Prepare vegetables, cutting into small uniform chunks. Add to large bowl and toss in olive, oil, salt and pepper. Gently toss in the rice, quinoa and couscous.

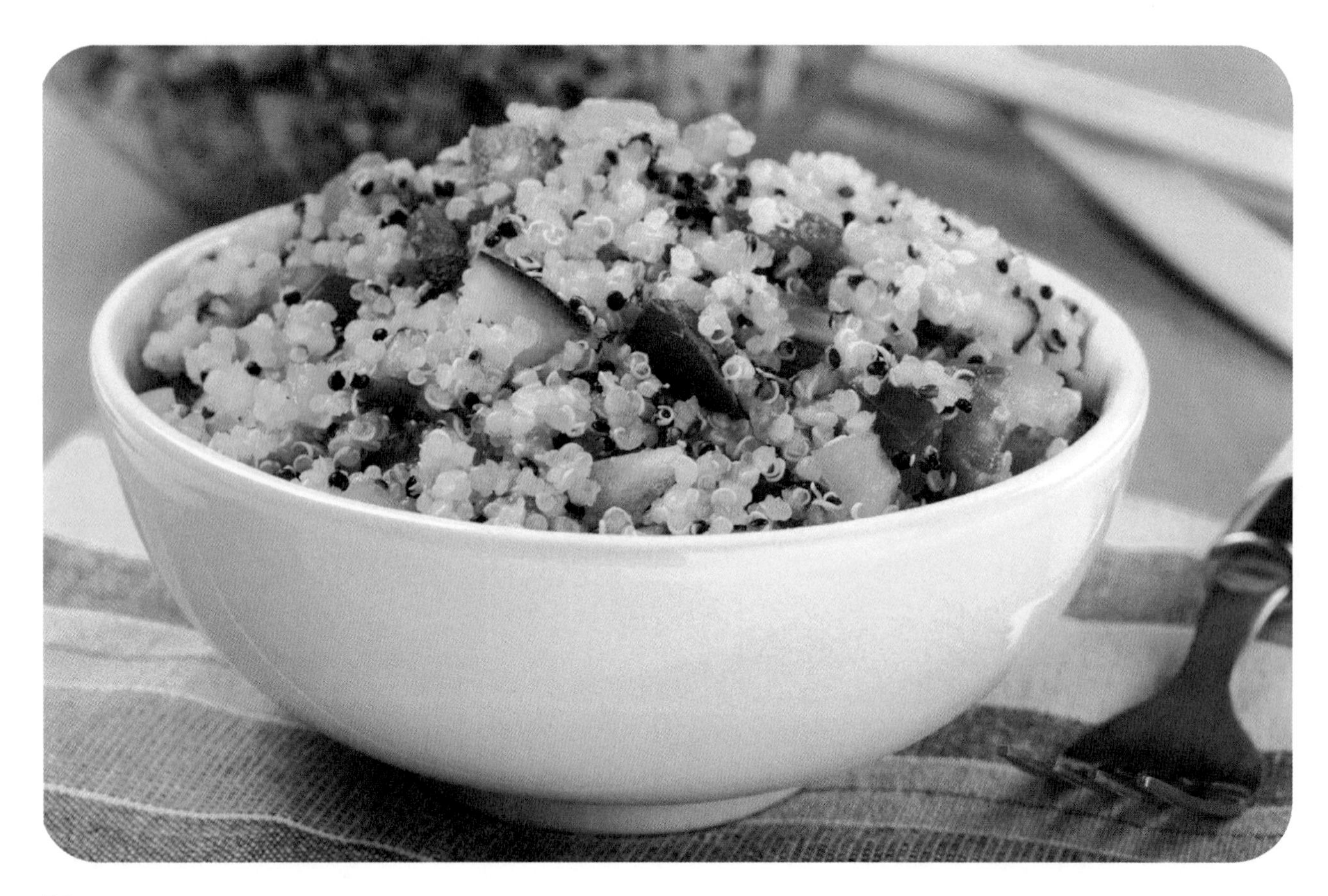

Pura Vida Morning Tonic

Pura Vida means "Livin' the good life, Livin' the dream." When we say, "Hello! How are you?" here in Costa Rica, we answer, "PURA VIDA!!"

Ingredients:

- 1 tsp each: cinnamon, turmeric, grated ginger
- ½ tsp cayenne pepper
- juice of 4 lemons
- 1 C kombucha
- water

Place ingredients in a pitcher. Stir and enjoy hot or iced throughout the day. I make it quite tart, so sometimes add stevia.

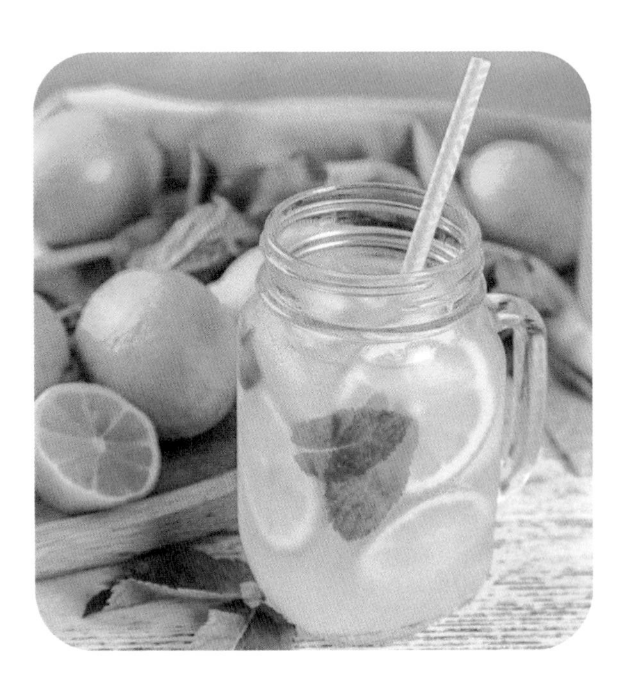

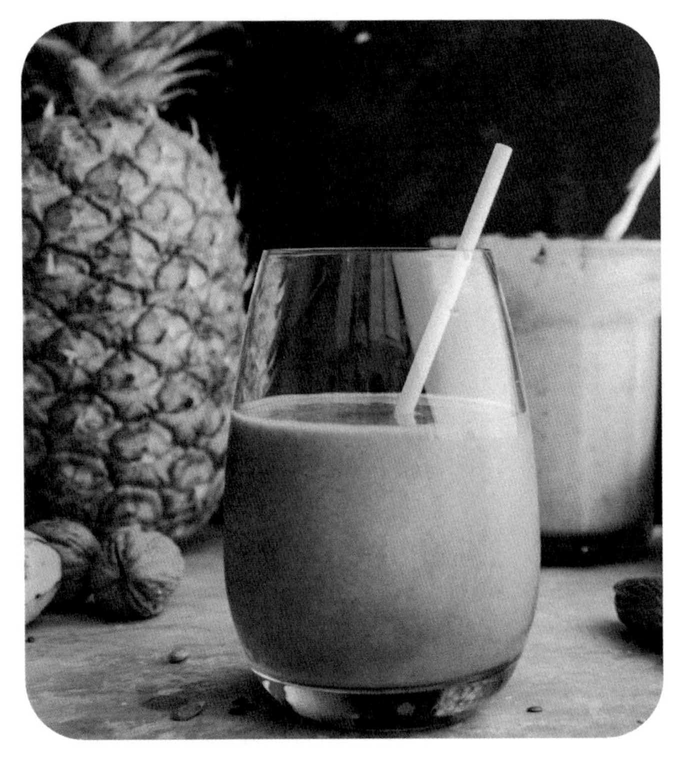

Pura Vida Morning Smoothie

Use the same base ingredients as above and add chopped pineapple, mango, papaya, avocado, kale, and/or banana.

I have all my fruit cut, divided, and frozen in zip lock bags. Each morning, I choose the "Sabor de Dia" ~ flavor of the day.

Hummus! Hummus! Hummus!

We love hummus and cook beans and chickpeas every day here on our retreat property, Paradiso Escondido, in Costa Rica. We like to create variations to keep it fun. Using hummus as the spread in wraps is bomb!

Basic Black Bean Hummus

Ingredients:

- 1½ C cooked black beans
- ¼ C tahini
- 2 cloves crushed garlic
- ½ C lemon juice
- water as needed
- salt and pepper
- pinch of cayenne pepper
- ½ tsp ground cumin

Put all ingredients in blender and whirl away! Add water as need. It should be a nice thick consistency. Serve with warm tortillas, pita bread, veggies and more.

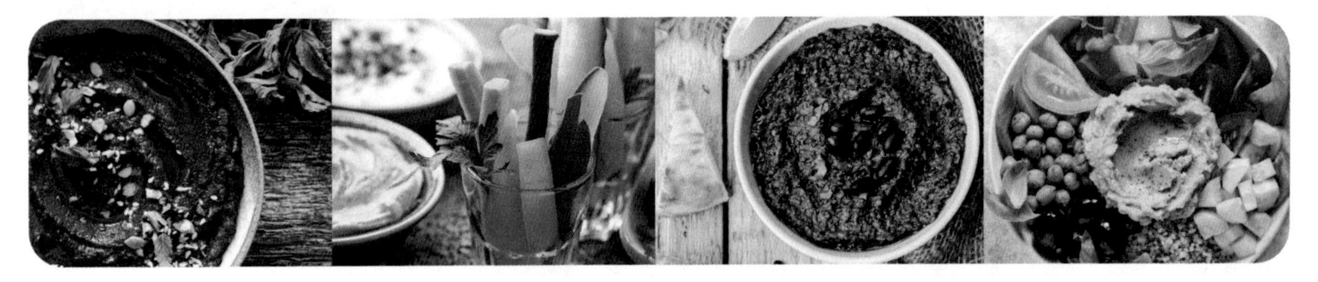

Beet Hummus

Start with the basic hummus recipe above. Omit the cumin. Add one boiled or roasted beet and ½ tsp dill. Blend well.

Creamy Vegan Cheesy Hummus

Start with the basic hummus recipe above. Substitute 1½ C cooked cannellini, white or lima beans for the black beans. Add ¼ C nutritional yeast. Blend well..

Green Goddess Hummus

Start with the basic hummus recipe above. Substitute 1½ C cooked chickpeas for the black beans. Add ½ C fresh herbs: basil, parsley, chives, cilantro + extra herbs to garnish. Blend well.

Pico de Gallo (Fresh Salsa)

Perfect for tacos, patacones (fried plantains), quesadillas or chips.

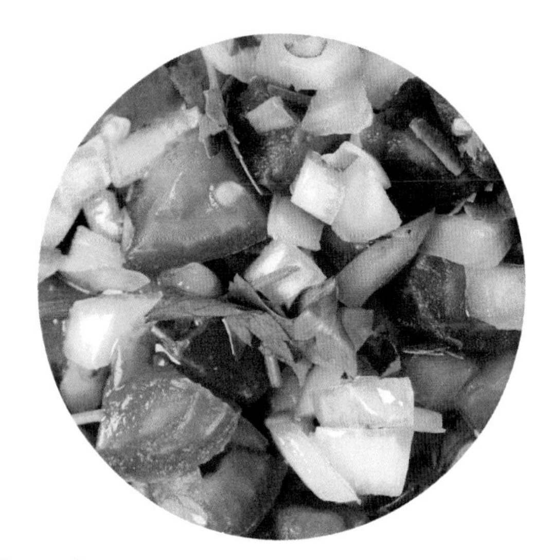

Ingredients:

- ¼ onion
- 2-3 medium tomatoes
- 1 jalapeño (remove ribs and seeds)
- ½ red bell pepper
- juice of 1 lime
- ½ C chopped cilantro
- oregano, cumin, salt and pepper to taste

To Prepare:

Cube all ingredients, place in serving bowl. Mix in spices, salt and pepper.

Mango Salsa

This sweet, sour, and spicy salsa is great on fish, patacones or chips.

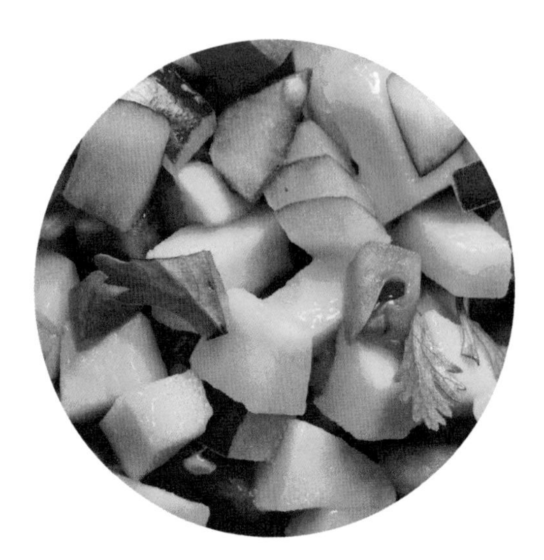

Ingredients:

- ¼ onion
- 2-3 medium tomatoes
- 1 jalapeño (remove ribs and seeds)
- ½ red bell pepper
- juice of 1 lime
- ½ C chopped cilantro
- oregano, cumin, salt and pepper to taste

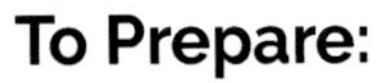

To Prepare:

Cube all ingredients, place in serving bowl. Mix in spices, salt and pepper.

Morning Glory Bread

The bread with options! What I love about this bread is you can interchange the fruits, vegetables and nuts. It's always amazingly healthy and can be prepared as muffins, mini-loaves, or in a traditional 9 x 13 inch pan.

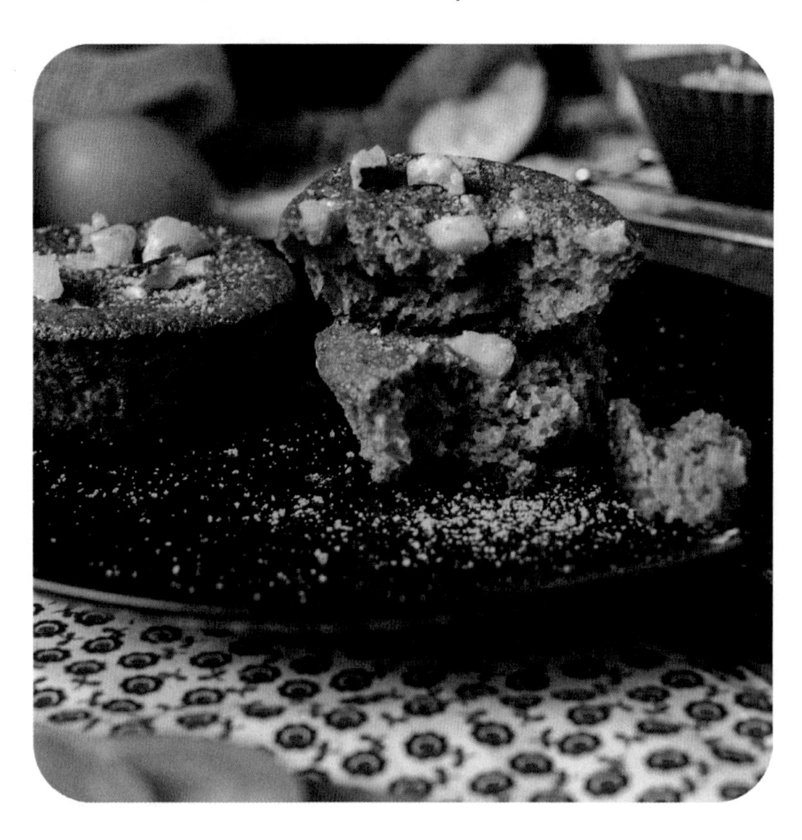

Ingredients:

- 2 C flour
- 1 ⅓ cups sugar
- 2 tsp baking soda
- 2 tsp cinnamon or pumpkin pie spice
- ½ C each: apple, zucchini, carrot, sweet potato
- 3 eggs
- ¾ C oil
- 1 tsp vanilla extract
- **Optional** - add to taste: raisins, shredded coconut, pecans

To Prepare:

Preheat oven to 350°F.

Mix dry and wet ingredients in separate bowls.

Then combine and transfer to greased 9 x 13" pan.

Bake for approximately 60 minutes, or until toothpick in center comes out clean. Adjust baking times as needed when using muffin pan or mini-loaves.

Rosemary Oil

For hair growth.

Ingredients:

- 5 rosemary sprigs
- 7 drops each of lavender, lemongrass, peppermint essential oils
- coconut, olive and avocado oils

To Prepare:

Cover rosemary sprigs in a heat-resistant glass or ceramic bowl with equal amounts of each oil.

In a large size saucepan, heat water to a boil, then turn down to low.

Place bowl with rosemary and oils (use glass bowl as double boiler) over saucepan and let heat for 30 minutes.

Strain rosemary, squeezing out all of the excess oil, being careful not to waste any.

Transfer to a jar or pump container.

Use weekly, massaging well into scalp and hair ends.

Cover hair with shower cap.

Shampoo after 20-30 minutes.

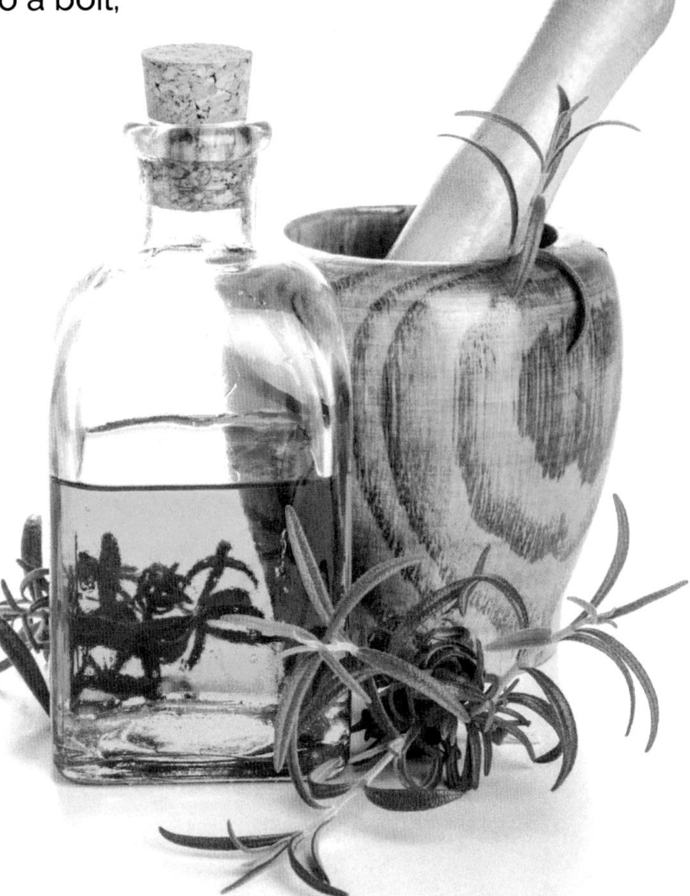

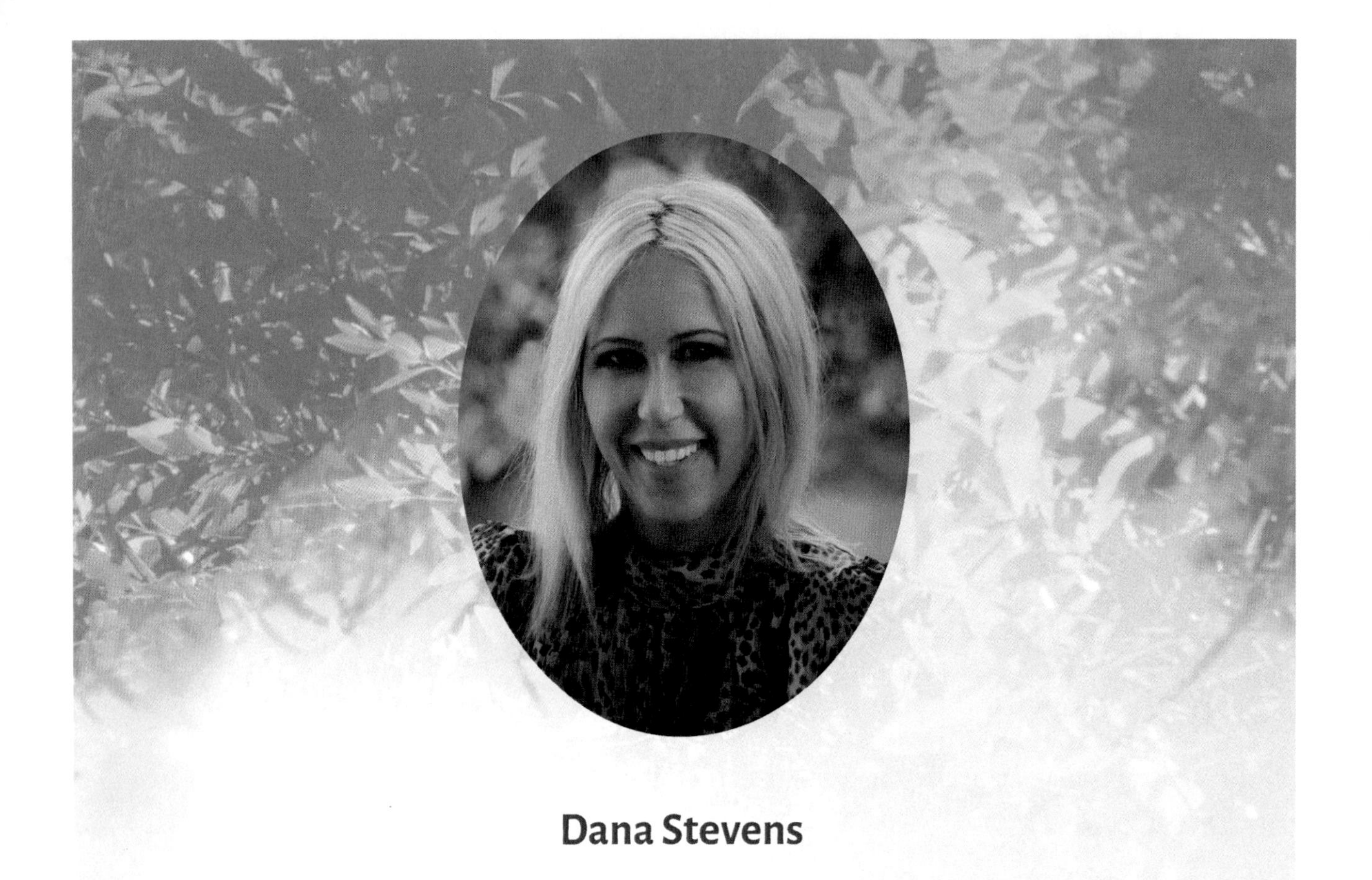

Dana Stevens

Dana Stevens began her real estate career in 2008 during the financial crisis. She was able to dive right in and experience what many agents had never encountered. Working with foreclosures and short sales only added to her resume. She has a background in construction by running a successful backhoe service with her husband. This lends itself to her extensive knowledge in the development of lots, moving homes, building and remodeling from the ground up. She uses her construction background to take a sophisticated approach when addressing her clients real estate needs.

Dana is always continuing her education to stay on top of the latest market trends, and technology. She obtained her Brokers License in order to represent her clients at the highest level.

As a longtime resident of Grass Valley, she has an intimate knowledge of Nevada County. When not traversing the Gold Country, you can find her mountain biking, hiking, playing pickleball, and enjoying all that the Foothills and Sierras have to offer.

Email: Danastevensrealtor@gmail.com

Summer Salad

Easy & delicious!

Ingredients:

- 1 can corn
- 2 avocados, diced
- 2 C tomatoes
- 1 cucumber, chopped
- ½ C crumbled feta
- ½ red onion, chopped

Viniagrette:

- 1 T rice vinegar
- 1 T white wine
- ½ tsp salt
- 1 tsp garlic powder
- 1 tsp garlic salt
- pepper, to taste
- basil, fresh, to taste
- splash of oil
- I add extra vinegar and just taste as I go

To Prepare:

Mix all ingredients for viniagrette.

Put all salad ingredients in a large bowl.

Add vinaigrette to taste.

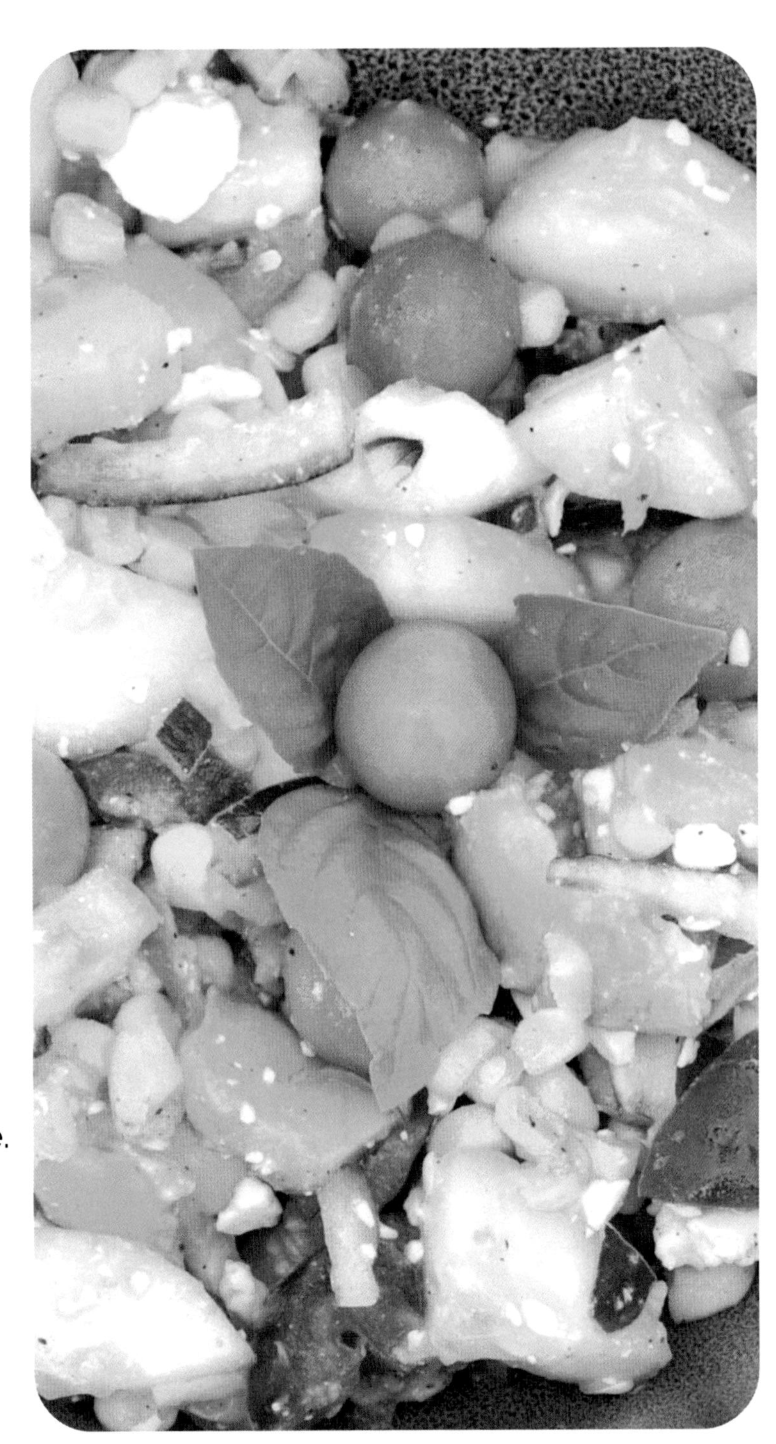

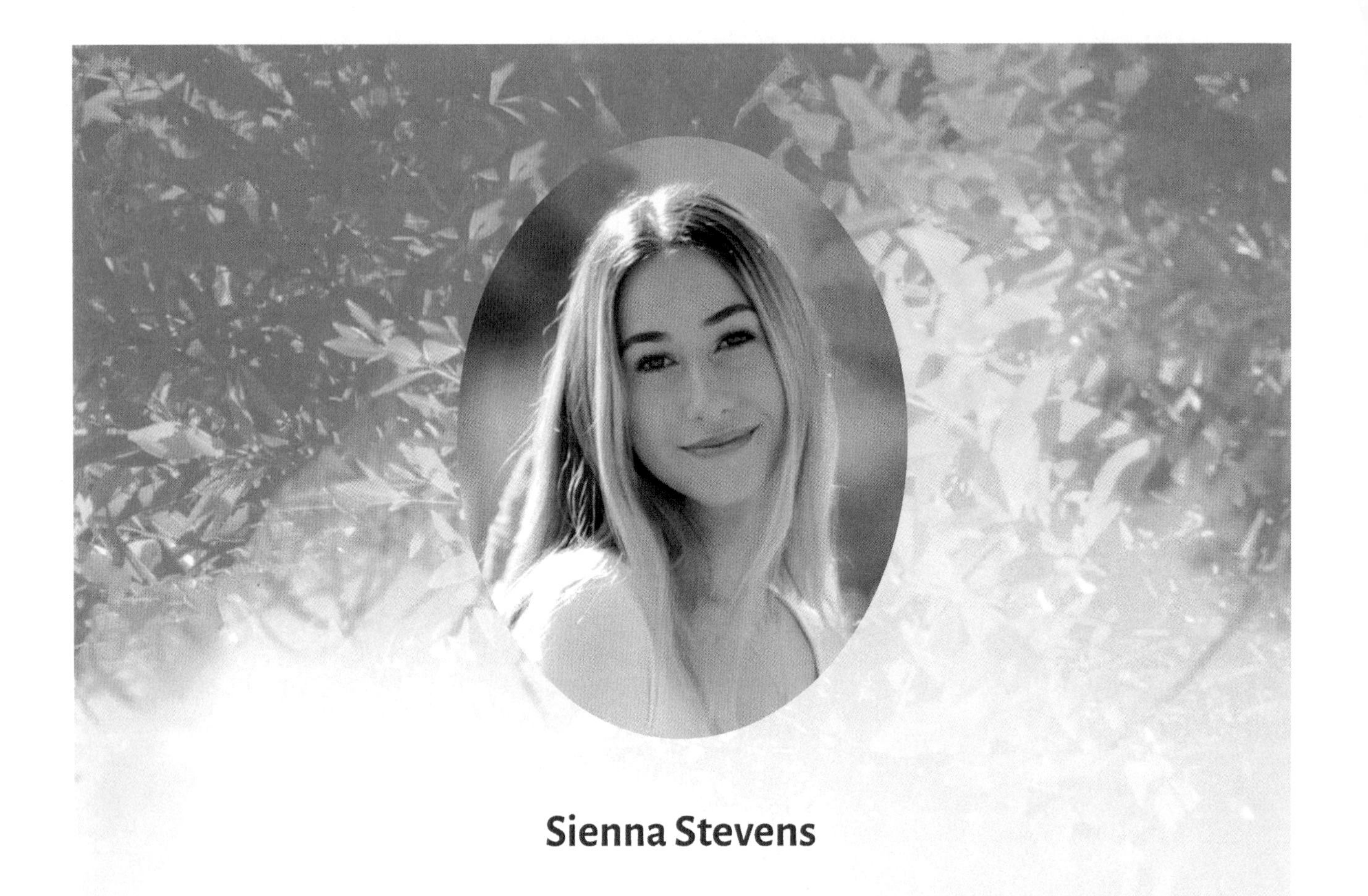

Sienna Stevens

Sienna Stevens is a tenacious young woman whose life took an unexpected turn when she was diagnosed with celiac disease at the age of 17. Her journey is a testament to her unwavering determination, resilience, and the transformative power of adapting to life's challenges.

The diagnosis of celiac disease meant that she had to bid farewell to her favorite gluten-containing foods and completely overhaul her diet. This transition was not without its difficulties. She faced the challenge of relearning how to shop for groceries, cook meals, and dine out, while ensuring her food was entirely gluten-free.

Rather than succumbing to despair, she embraced the challenge. Sienna embarked on a culinary adventure: exploring gluten-free recipes, experimenting with alternative ingredients, and mastering the art of gluten-free cooking. Her kitchen became a haven of creativity, where she transformed her favorite dishes into gluten-free delights. This recipe is one of her favorites, and she encourages you to use all gluten-free ingredients.

No Bake Chocolate Chip Oatmeal Bars

I have struggled with Celiac Disease and so these bars have been a perfect snack for me. I use all gluten-free ingredients when I make them, and it turns out delicious!

Ingredients:

- 1 C smooth organic nut butter
- ⅔ C local honey
- 1 tsp vanilla
- ½ tsp salt
- 2 ½ C oats
- ⅓ C mini chocolate chips
- ¼ C chopped nuts optional (your choice)

To Prepare:

Stir together nut butter, honey, vanilla, and salt until smooth. Add oats, chocolate chips and nuts.

Place in an 8 x 8 inch pan which is lined with parchment paper. Place another piece of parchment paper on top and press down firmly to flatten.

Chill for 1 hour and cut into squares. Enjoy.

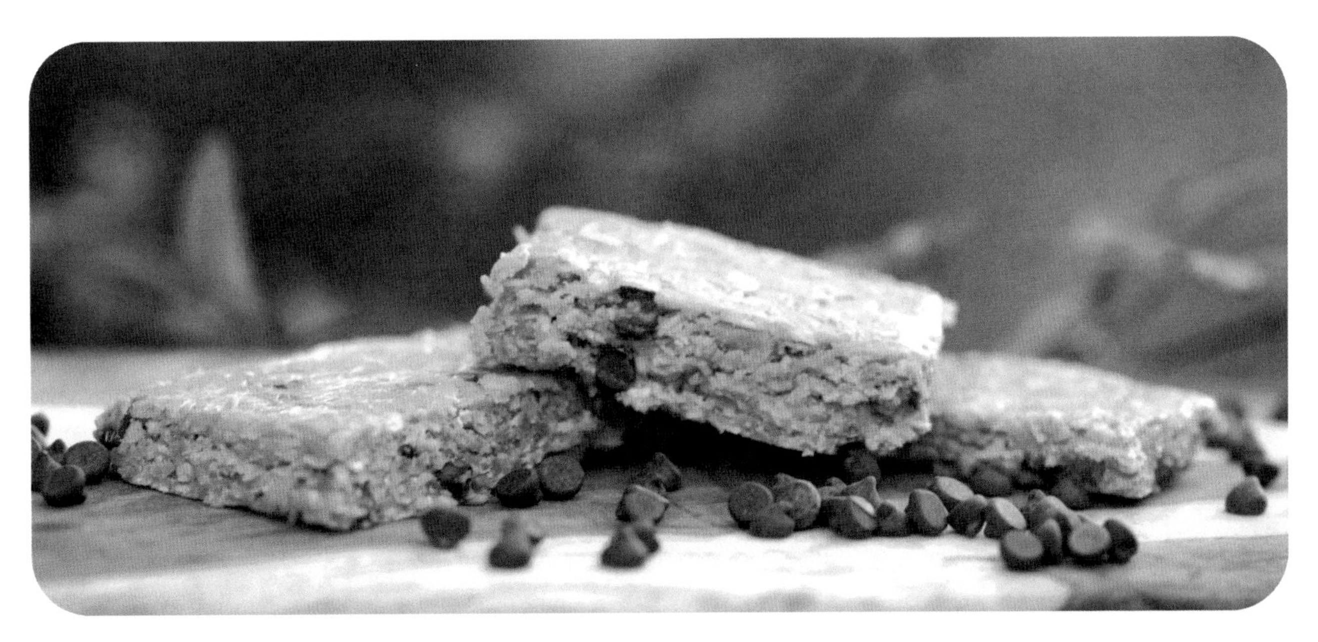

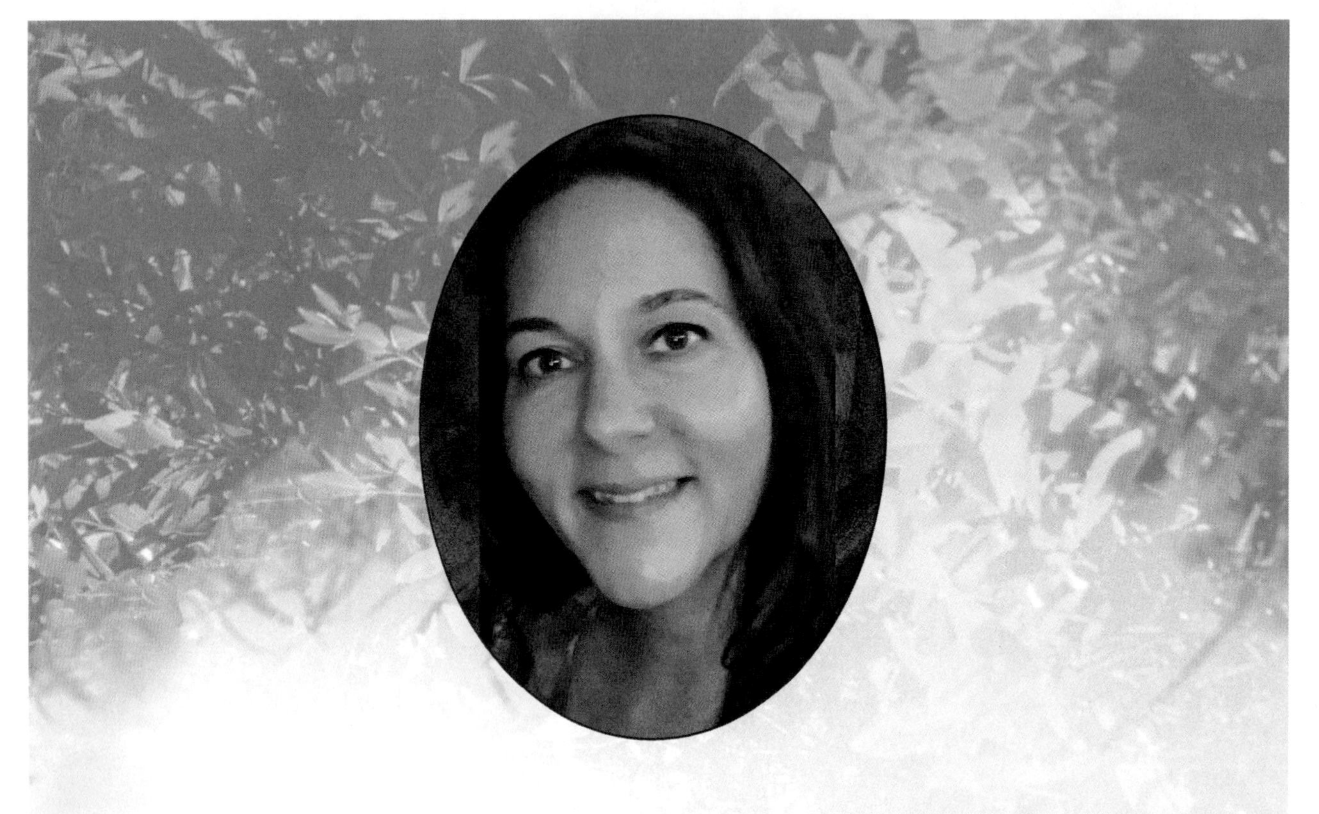

GINA VIAN

Gina is a mother of two boys, an elementary school teacher, a lover of all things outdoors, and always up for adventures. She loves to travel and spend time with her boys and her friends and family.

Her passion for cooking and baking started at a young age when she spent time in the kitchen making delicious meals and desserts with her mother. She continues to enjoy baking as an adult, with her sons.

Now she has taken on the challenge of creating healthy dishes and modifying traditionally unhealthy meals to make them healthier. "I have always had a sweet tooth, but it is important to me to live a healthy lifestyle, so it has been my mission to create foods that satisfy my sweet tooth but are also clean and healthier for my boys and me."

Chocolate Chocolate Muffins

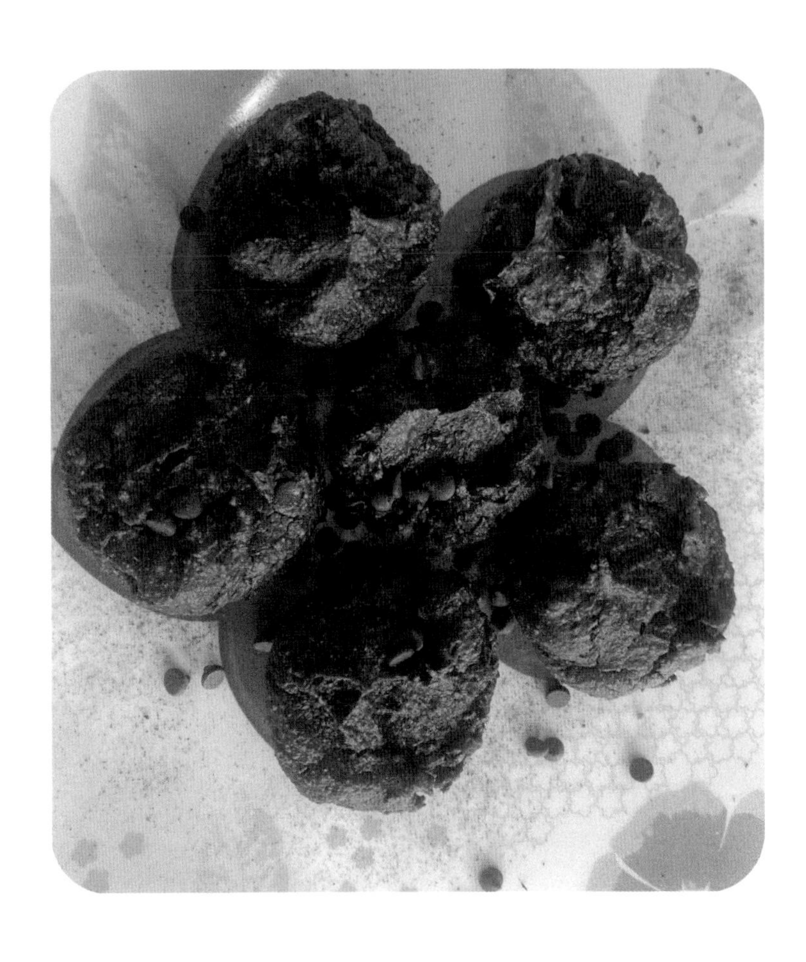

Ingredients:

- 2 large eggs
- ½ C organic maple syrup
- 1 ½ C organic pumpkin puree
- 2 tsp vanilla extract
- 2 C organic peanut butter or almond butter
- 6 T unsweetened cacao powder
- 2 tsp baking soda
- 1 tsp cinnamon
- ½-¾ C cacao, or dark chocolate chips

To Prepare:

Mix all wet ingredients first.

Mix the cacao powder with the baking soda and cinnamon and then mix in with the wet ingredients.

Grease a muffin pan and fill muffin tins ¾ full of the mixture.

Bake at 350°F for 15-20 minutes.

> TIP: I take my muffins out when there is just a little bit of the mixture on the toothpick. I find if I wait until the toothpick comes out clean, the muffins turn out too dry.

Clean Chocolate Peanut Butter Bites

Ingredients:

- 1 C low sugar dark chocolate chips
- ¼-⅓ C organic peanut or almond butter
  (Room temperature works best.)

To Prepare:

Melt the chocolate chips in the microwave or on the stove. Stir frequently.

Once the chocolate is melted, mix in the peanut or almond butter and pour into a muffin tin. Fill each cup ¼ full. You can also use a mini muffin pan for smaller bites.

Protein Date Balls

Ingredients:

- 2 C Medjool dates, pitted
- 2 C almonds (or other nuts/seeds)
- 1 C shredded, unsweetened coconut
- 1 tsp vanilla extract
- 1 tsp cinnamon (optional)

To Prepare:

Soak dates in warm water for at least 10 minutes, then drain. Put all ingredients in a food processor until all are broken down and crumbly. Mixture will start to form a ball.

Once the mixture is ready, use a spoon to scoop the mixture and form into balls.

Protein date balls can be kept in the refrigerator or stored in the freezer.

Energy Balls

These are perfect for a quick breakfast, snack, or even as a healthy dessert option.

Ingredients:

- 1 ½ C organic almond butter or peanut butter
- ⅔ C organic maple syrup or honey
- 2 tsp vanilla extract
- 2 C gluten-free rolled oats (uncooked)
- 2-4 scoops vanilla or chocolate protein powder
- 1 C freeze dried strawberries
- ⅔ C dark chocolate chips/cacao (optional)
- 4 T chopped almonds (optional)
- 2 tsp cinnamon (optional)

To Prepare:

Combine wet ingredients first. Mix in dry ingredients. With your hands, form into 1 inch balls. Keep refrigerated.

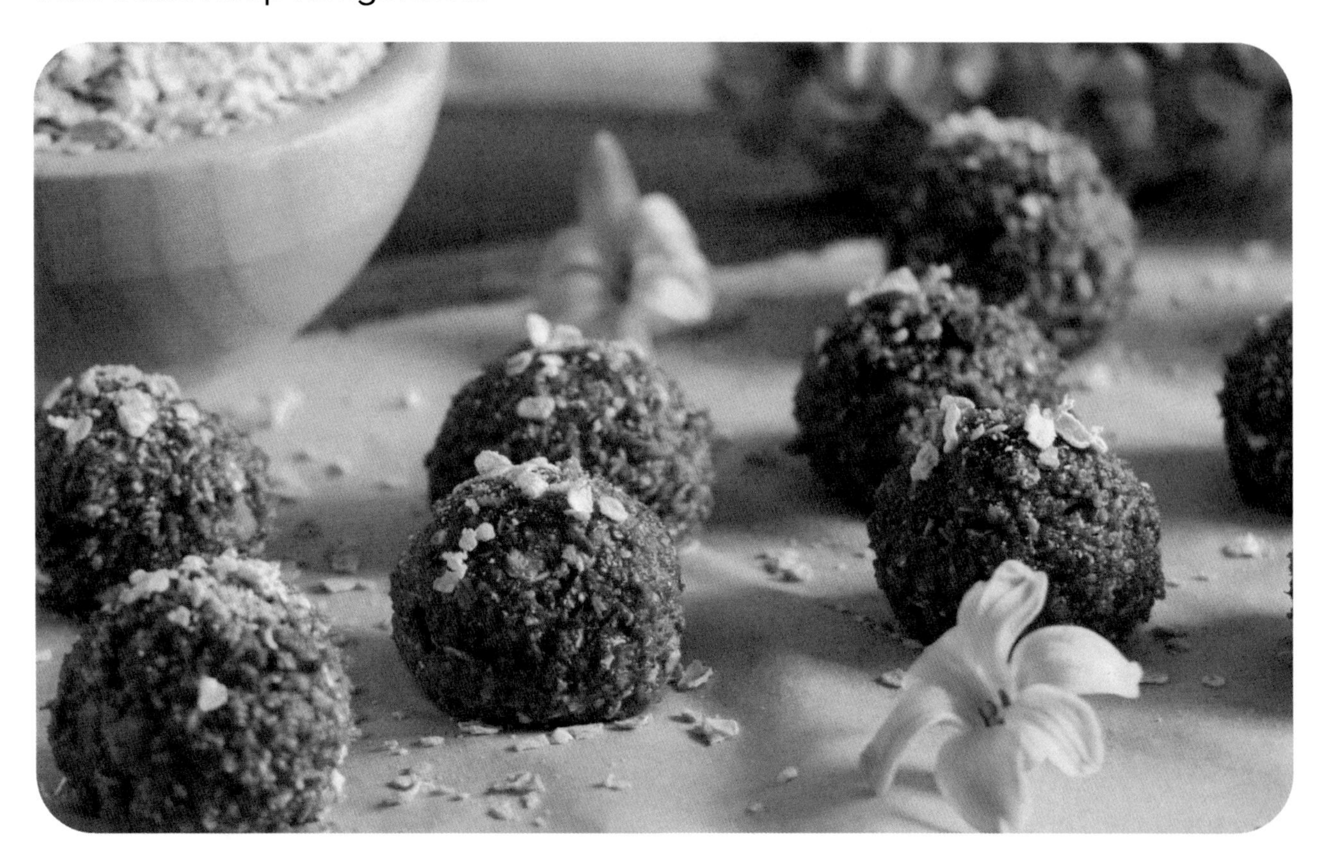

Pumpkin Spice Smoothie

Ingredients:

- 1 frozen ripe banana
- ½ C unsweetened almond milk or coconut milk
- 1 C pumpkin puree
- 2 T organic almond butter or peanut butter
- ¼ tsp ground cinnamon
- ¼ tsp pumpkin pie spice
- 1 C ice cubes

To Prepare:

Put all ingredients in a blender and blend until smooth.

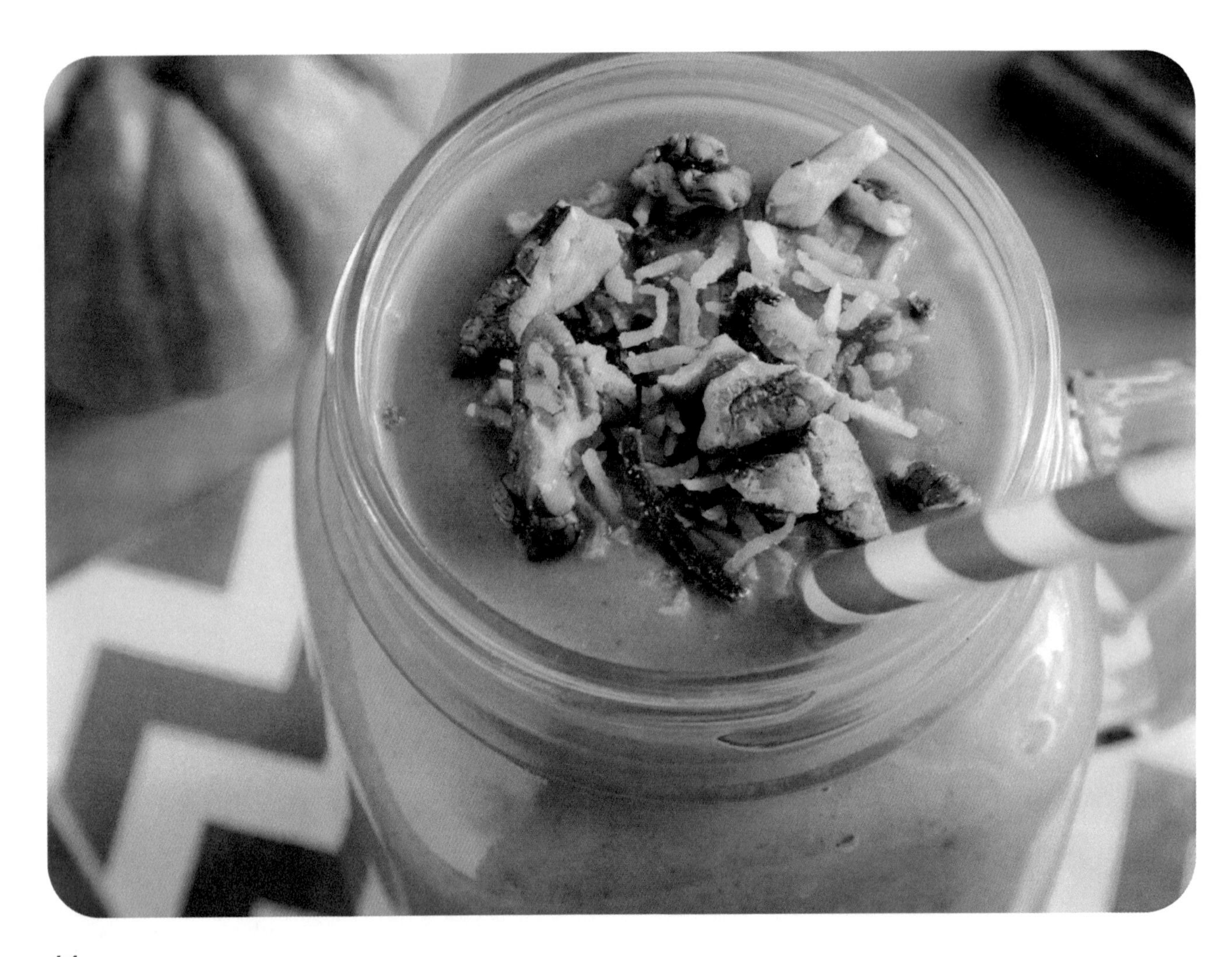

Pineapple Frozen Delight

A perfect refreshing dessert for a hot summer evening.

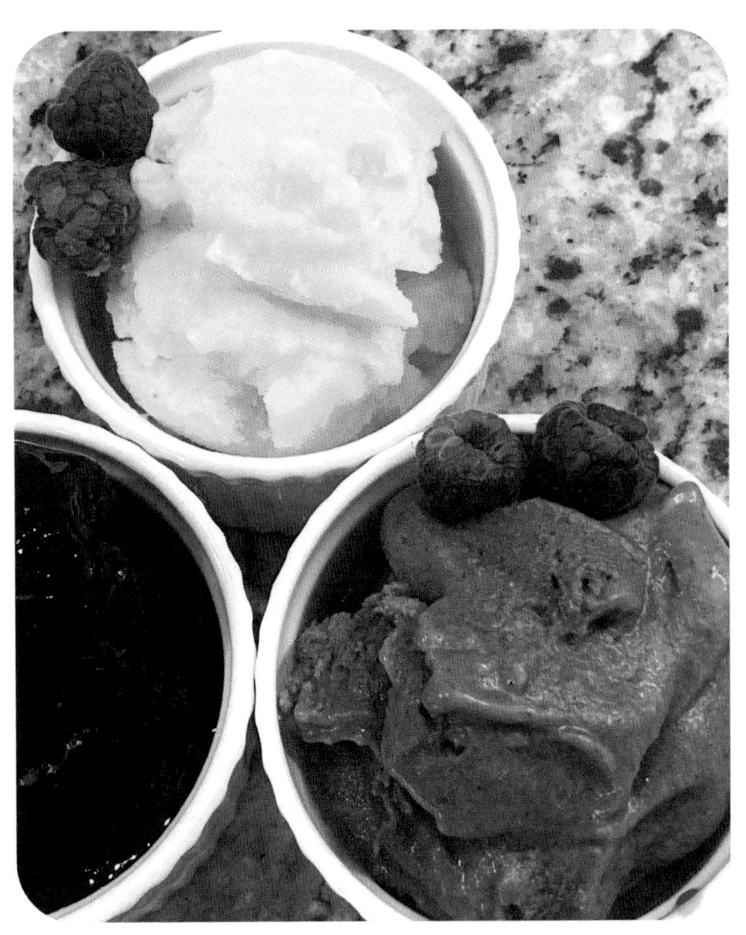

Ingredients:

- 4-5 C frozen organic pineapple chunks
- ½-¾ C organic, unsweetened coconut milk

To Prepare:

Allow frozen pineapple to sit out for a few minutes to thaw just a little bit.

Put pineapple chunks in the blender and add coconut milk. Add more or less depending on the consistency you like.

Cherry Nice Cream

Ingredients:

- 4-5 C frozen cherries
- ½-¾ C organic, unsweetened coconut milk
- 3 T organic almond butter
  (optional, but it gives this nice cream a nutty flavor)

To Prepare:

Allow frozen cherries to sit out for a few minutes to thaw just a little bit.

Put cherries in the blender and add coconut milk and almond butter.

Blend to desired consistency.

Berry Oatmeal Muffins

Ingredients:

- 2 ripe bananas
- ⅓ C organic maple syrup
- 3 large eggs
- ½ T vanilla extract
- 1 C unsweetened coconut or almond milk
- 2 C rolled oats
- ½ C coconut or almond flour
- 1 tsp cinnamon (optional)
- 1 ½ tsp baking powder
- 1 C mixed berries

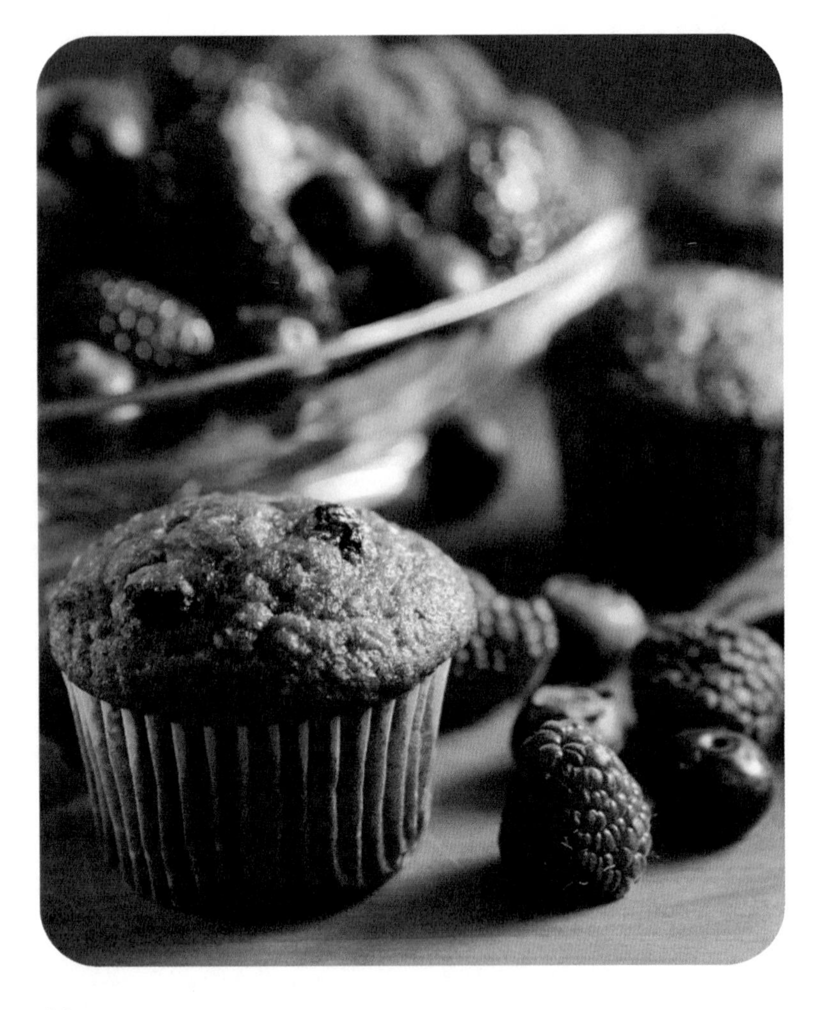

To Prepare:

Preheat oven to 350°F.

Place bananas in a bowl and mash them with a fork. Add the rest of the wet ingredients and mix.

Add all of the dry ingredients and mix well.

Gently fold in the berries.

Lightly spray a muffin tray with olive or coconut oil. Fill each muffin cup ⅔ full.

Bake in preheated oven for 15-17 minutes, or until a toothpick inserted into the center comes out clean.

Oatmeal Bake

You can swap out the zucchini and chocolate chips for shredded carrots and raisins, or unsweetened coconut and dried cranberries.

Ingredients:

- 1 C coconut or unsweetened almond milk
- 2 T coconut oil, melted
- 2 eggs
- 3 C gluten-free quick cooking oats
- ½ C coconut sugar
- 2 tsp baking powder
- 1 tsp cinnamon
- 2 tsp vanilla
- 1 ½ C grated zucchini (Pat the zucchini dry prior to mixing in.)
- ½ C chocolate chips (optional)

To Prepare:

Preheat oven to 350°F.

In a large bowl combine wet ingredients first and then add the dry ingredients.

Stir in the zucchini and then fold in the chocolate chips (or alternate ingredients.)

Spread mixture evenly into a greased 9 x 13 inch pan and bake for 20-25 minutes, depending on the consistency that you like.

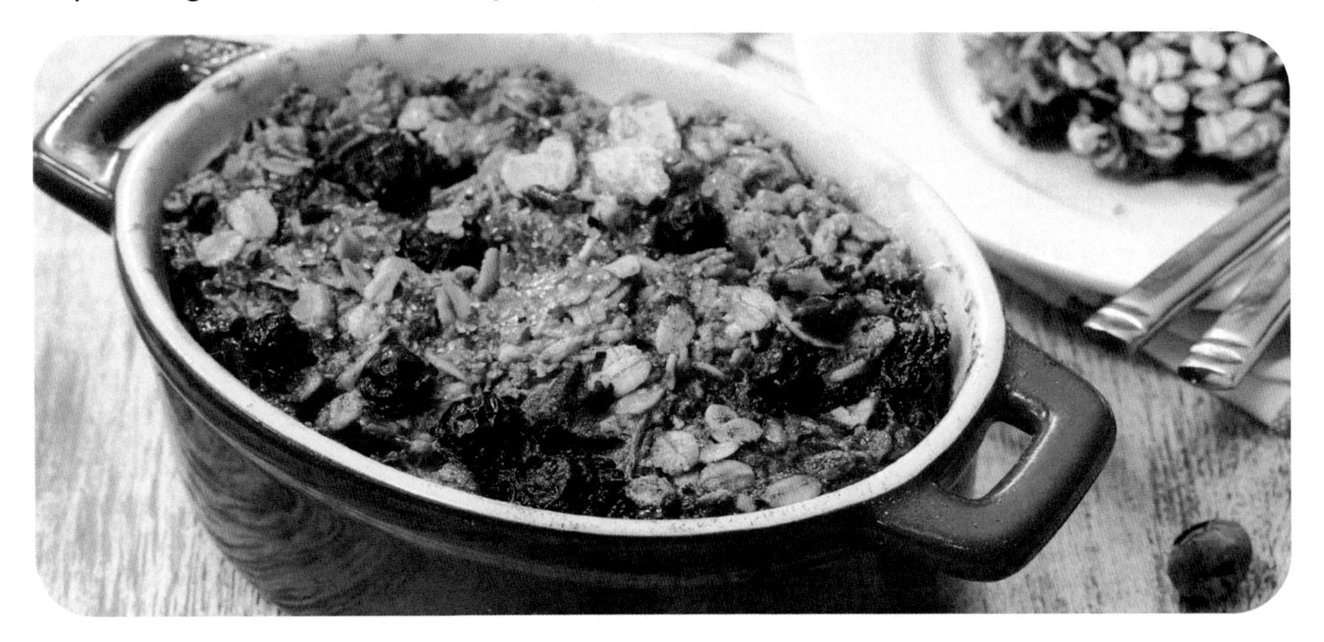

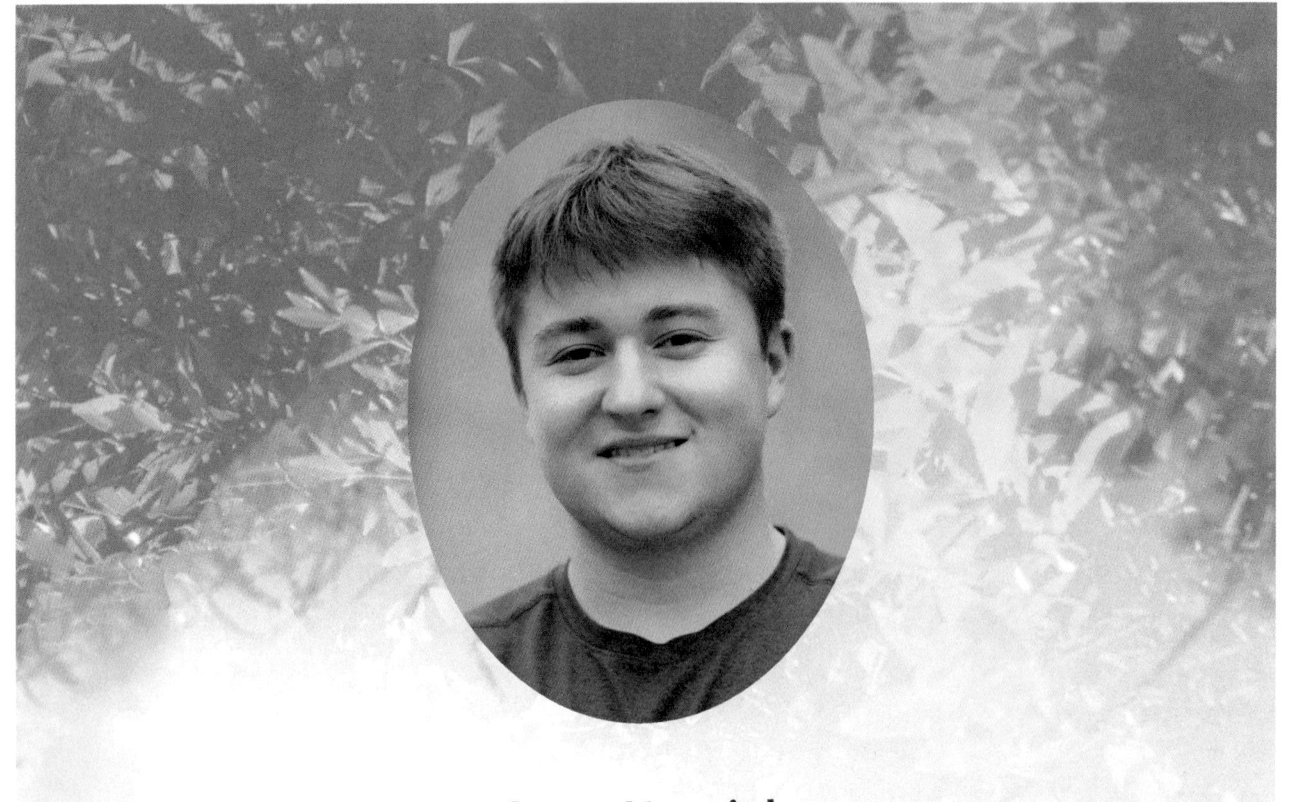

Carter Nunnink

Carter Nunnink's desire to create the best organic Peanut Butter Chocolate Chip cookies comes from within his soul. Carter was born in 2004 with an innate desire to be the best at anything he sets his mind to, whether playing basketball, doing schoolwork, or cooking. Carter learned to cook by watching his mom and dad cook healthy recipes at home. In addition, he began watching YouTube cooking videos a few years ago, which led to the creation of the simple Organic Peanut Butter Chocolate Chip cookie recipe. These cookies quickly became a smash hit with his family and have earned them the nickname "Killer Cookies." Carter's other favorite things to cook for his family are Chicken Alfredo and fajitas. For Christmas 2022, Carter received an ice cream maker and enjoys making many different ice cream flavors by modifying a basic recipe. The current family favorite is Chocolate Mint, which uses gluten-free Oreo mint cookie crumbles.

In addition to cooking, Carter enjoys playing recreational basketball with his friends. Currently he is attending Sierra College in Grass Valley, California, with plans to transfer to a university in the fall of 2024.

Gluten-free Peanut Butter Chocolate Chip Cookies

Gluten-free & protein rich! Use organic ingredients.

Ingredients:

- 1 C brown sugar
- 1 egg
- 1 C peanut butter
- 1 C chocolate chips
- 1 tsp baking soda

To Prepare:

Roll dough in balls and place on a baking sheet lined with parchment paper. Use a fork to make criss-cross designs and flatten each dough ball.

Bake at 400°F for approximately 6-7 minutes or until done.

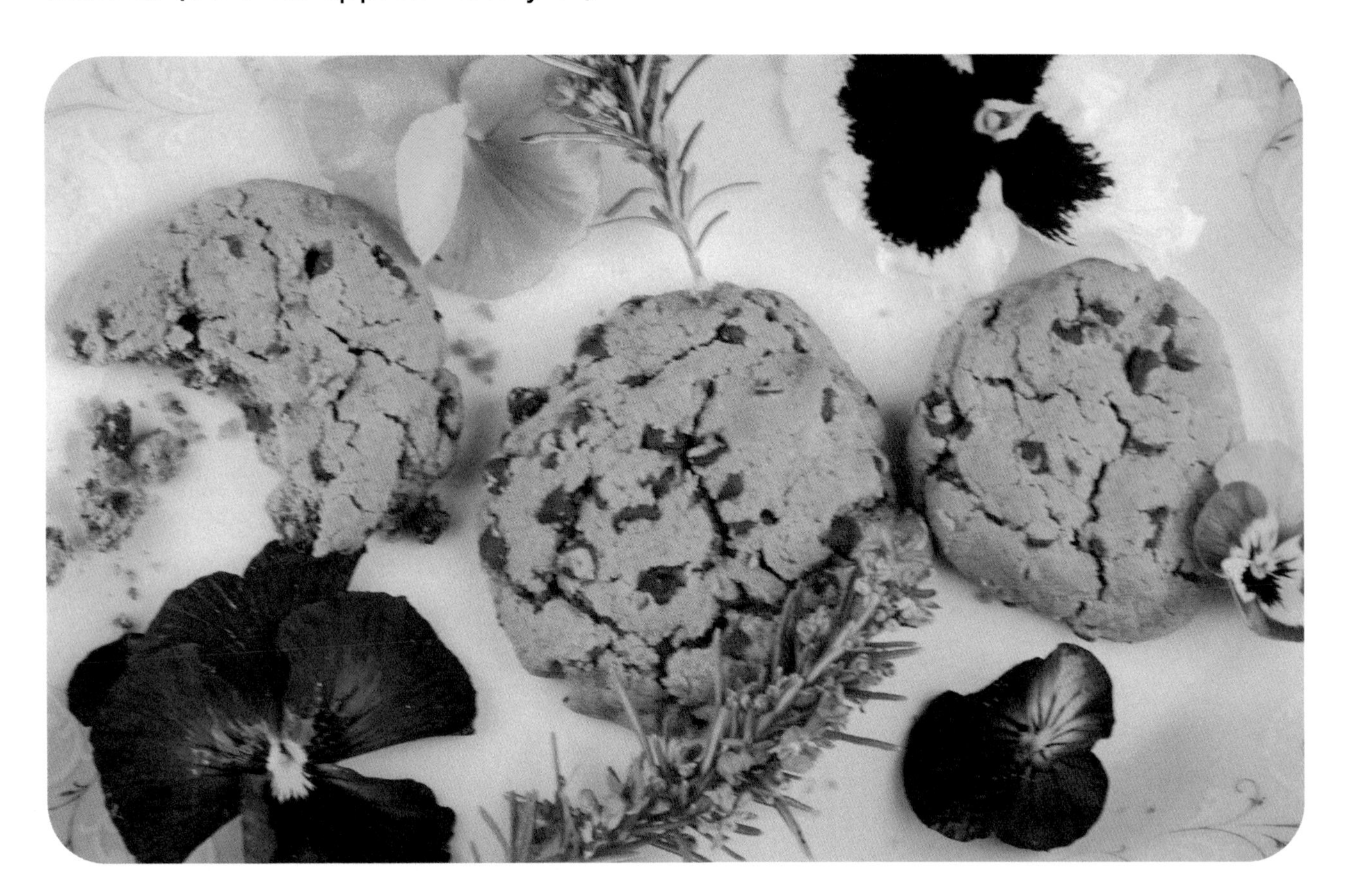

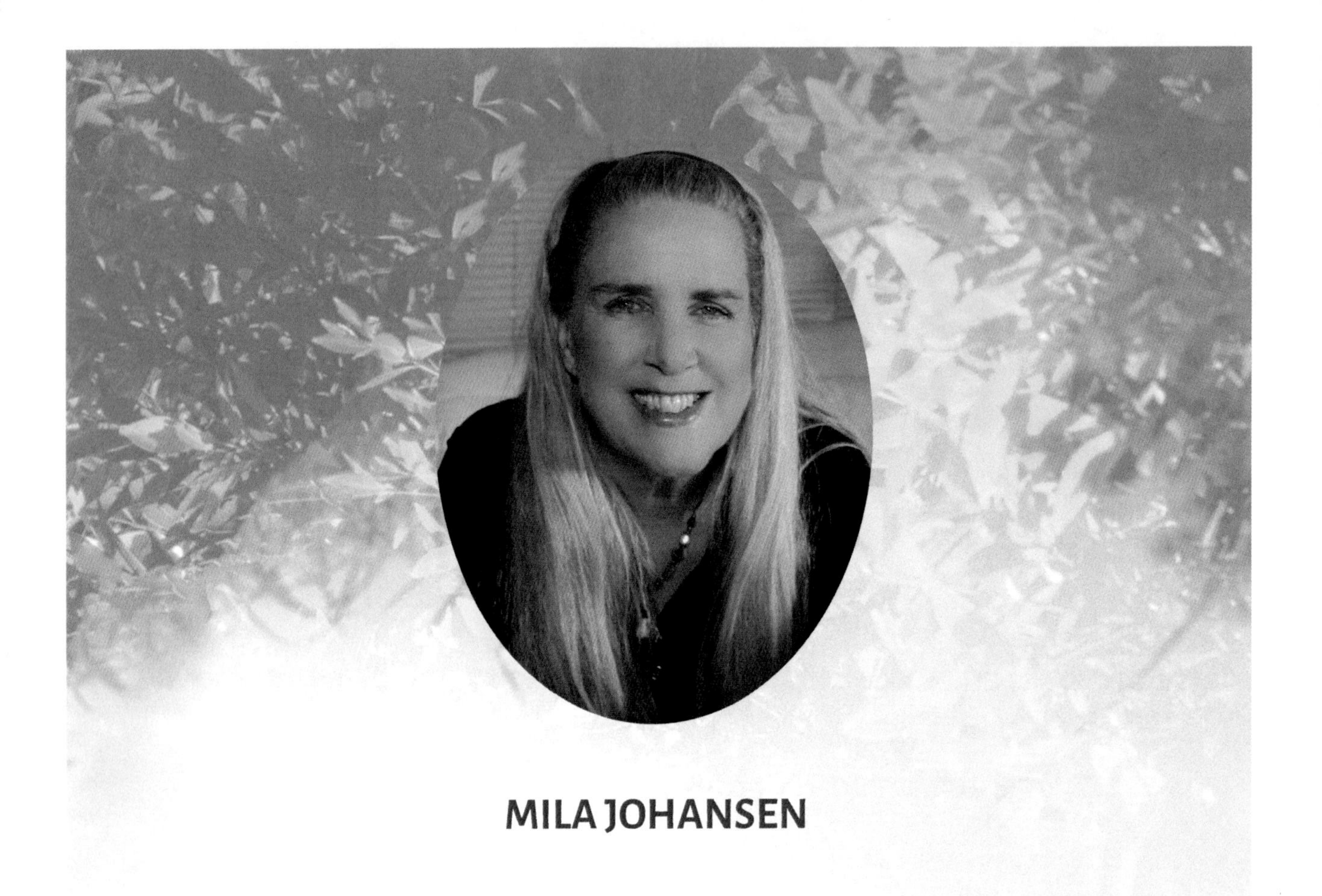

MILA JOHANSEN

Mila Johansen is a public speaker, writing and publishing coach, teacher, and writer. She is the best-selling author of nine books, including *From Cowgirl to Congress: Journey of a Suffragist on the Front Lines.* This is a first-person account from Jessie Haver Butler, Mila's grandmother. who was the first woman lobbyist in D.C. and taught public speaking to Eleanor Roosevelt. Mila also has several more books in progress and loves to write and produce short screenplays. She has developed "The Short Book" concept giving people all over the world permission to write their "short book" first.

Mila lives on an organic ranch with her husband and three dogs. She grew up near Los Angeles and thought mandarins grew in a can. She attended college at Chico State, where she met her husband. He put her to work on his organic citrus ranch. She soon found herself running the entire harvest by herself: hiring and running the packing crew, loading semis with a forklift, and loving every minute of it.

Email: johansenmila@gmail.com
Website: milajohansen.com

9

Thanksgiving With A Twist

Mila Johansen

"Food for the body is not enough.
There must be food for the soul."

~ Dorothy Day

I grew up in a single-parent household. My mother was a grade school teacher, but the salary barely covered expenses. I remember going to bed many nights without dinner. I remember going to school and watching the other kids feast on sack lunches while I went without. But please do not feel sorry for me, I married an organic citrus farmer and never went hungry again. I always wondered why the trees on my college campuses were not fruit trees to feed all of us starving students. Because of my upbringing in poverty, my husband and I donate more than 10,000 pounds of citrus a year to our local food banks.

My mother had to rise in the mornings at 5 a.m. and leave the house by 6 a.m. to drive the 45 minutes to her teaching job in the next county. She had a weak constitution, so would get home around 5 o'clock in the evening and go to her room to sleep. That left me with all the housework, cooking, and care of my younger brother from about the age of 10. I had to make him breakfast, get him out the door to walk to school, and make him dinner when he came home—and do all the housework. For years, I was a real Cinderella. I have to say, that all that responsibility gave me a tremendous work ethic that has served me all my life. When I met my husband, Rich, he put me to work on the citrus ranch, and boy, did he luck out. I worked 8-12 hour days and hardly ever complained. I actually thrived.

My mother did cook for us occasionally. Every Sunday, she would make a roast dinner with potatoes and carrots and it was delicious. That was before I became what

I call a "red meat vegetarian" in college. Chicken was half the price of red meat. So, that summer when I ate a roast beef sandwich, I doubled over in pain from not eating red meat for the previous year. After that, I never ate it again. The irony is, I married into the last remaining slaughterhouse in Northern California and we just recently inherited part of it. Yikes! I haven't had red meat in 47 years—and I am so glad about that.

My mother also cooked on all the holidays. Confession. My meals as a young girl often consisted of macaroni from a box and Rice-a-Roni. Our favorite was when I served "make your own tacos." I would set out grated cheese, crumbled fried hamburger, lettuce, and other ingredients and then we would both make our own tacos. It is still the favorite for my daughter, husband and me (but now we use ground turkey).

As I grew older, I began to look up recipes and extend my repertoire. I began baking 3-layer lemon cakes. What made me famous with friends were the chocolate chip cookies I would make whenever we went on camping trips, which was often. I would bake so many that I had to carry them in large, paper shopping bags.

My mother always made huge Thanksgiving dinners. It would wear her out, but she did it. I remember as a teenager when she handed the Thanksgiving baton to me. From then on, I made all of the Thanksgiving dinners, and still do for our family today. I have included many of my favorite recipes in this book. It's a non-traditional Thanksgiving, however, as we feast on both turkey and nut loaf.

I told my husband before we were married that I might never cook, just to stop any expectations. He said, "That's fine, my mother didn't always cook." Of course, I do cook, about two to three times a week. I hardly ever make a meal for just one night; I prepare a casserole, or quinoa salad, or soup that we can enjoy all week. I usually make two or three items, like a pot of beans, a big salad, and muffins. I often follow in my mother's cooking footsteps and make a giant roasted chicken dinner with potatoes and carrots that we can enjoy all week.

In fact, I have been working on my own cookbook for the past 40 years. It's called *Cook on Monday—Eat 'til Sunday*. Look for it on Amazon. It's jam-packed with recipes you can cook once and eat from all week and . . . follow in *my* footsteps.

Sugared Sage

On my herbal summer tour with Kathi Keville in Italy, we were served sage fronds in a very light tempura batter. When I came home and saw all the sage growing on my organic farm, I picked a bunch, looked up some recipes online and tried out several versions. These two are the best of the recipes that I adapted and are amazingly delicious! Serve them at Thanksgiving or parties. They make wonderful after-dinner treats.

Ingredients:

- freshly picked sage, in 4-6" sprigs - including stems with leaves
- olive or avocado oil spray
- sugar, preferably organic

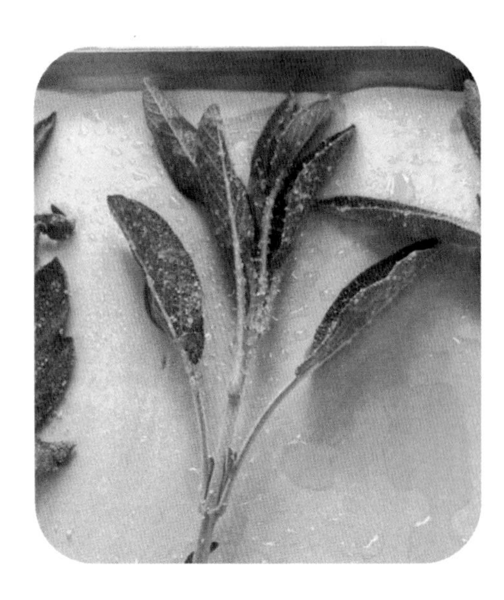

Holding each sprig by the stem, fan out the leaves. Lightly spray them with olive or avocado oil. Spraying makes coverage more even.

Hold each sprig over a bowl and pinch sugar between index finger and thumb to sprinkle over every part of the surface on both sides.

Using a non-stick or lined with parchment paper cookie sheet, lay out the sugared pieces. Heat in the oven at 250°F for about 20-30 minutes, until stiff and crunchy.

Tempura Sage Fronds

Ingredients:

- freshly picked sage, in 4-6" sprigs - including stems with leaves
- Pamela's Gluten-free Flour (or flour of your choice)
- mango, or other fruit juice
- honey or sugar, to taste

Make a light tempura batter by blending flour and a bit of fruit juice. Add sweetener as desired. Experiment with flavors and consistency. Swirl each sage frond in the batter, letting any extra batter drip back into bowl.

Using a non-stick or lined with parchment paper cookie sheet, lay out the sugared pieces. Heat in the oven at 250°F for about 20-30 minutes, until stiff and crunchy.

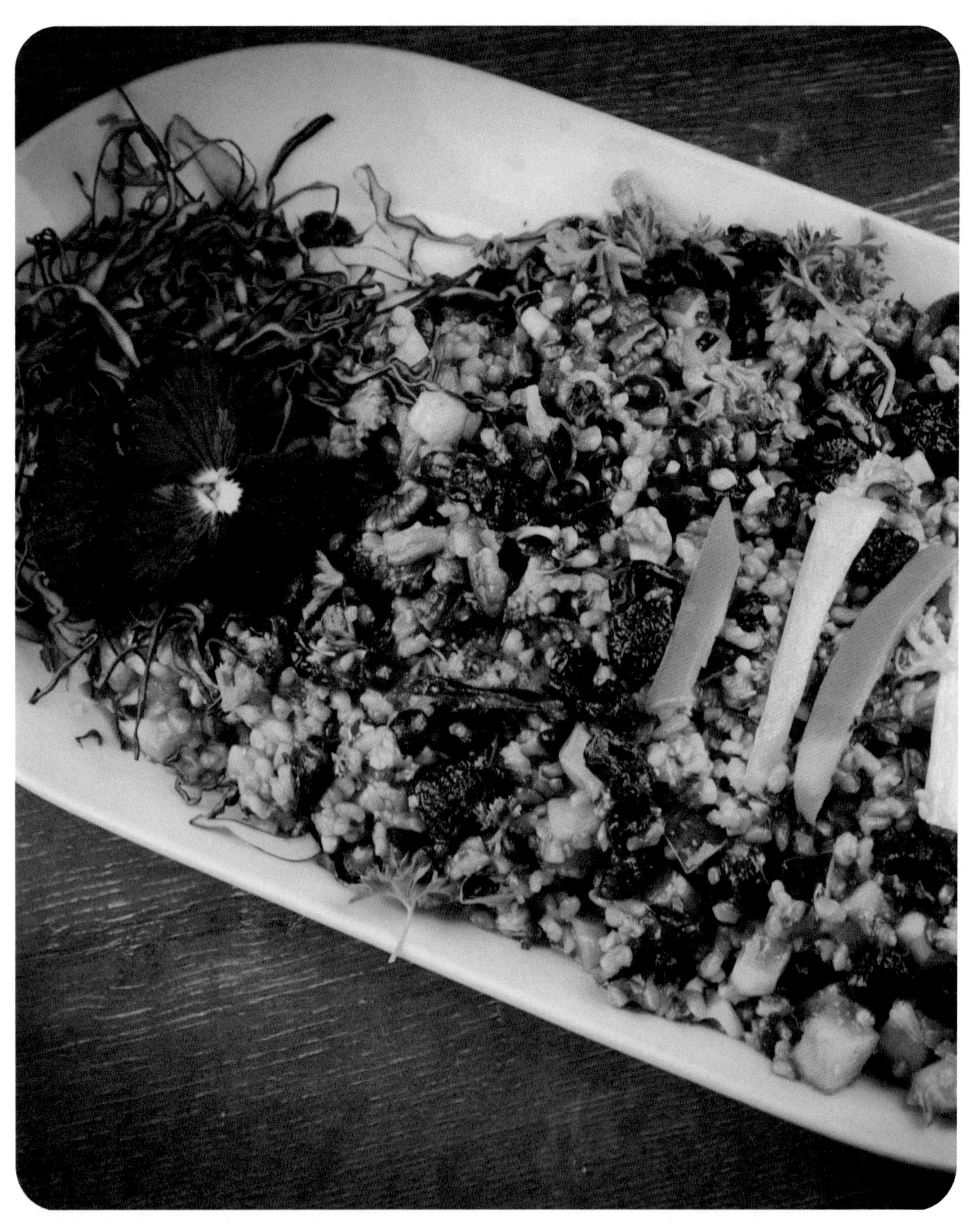

The Spice of Life Rice Salad

Pre-cook:

- 2 C short-grain brown rice in 4C water (2-to-1); any grain can be used
- Add a pinch of salt.
- Don't overcook the rice. Let rice cool.

Pre-soak:

- ½ C+ raisins or currants, to taste

While rice is cooking, chop very finely in a food processor (or with knife):

- 1 bunch parsley
- 4-5 carrots
- 4-5 celery stalks
- ¼ head red cabbage
- ½ bunch broccoli
- ½ C or more walnuts or almonds

Dice a good amount of tofu or feta cheese.

Mix everything in a large bowl and add (more or less):

- 1-3 T balsamic vinegar
- 1 tsp or more salt
- ⅓ C tamari or soy sauce
- ¼ C or more honey
- 1 T lemon juice
- 1 tsp brown mustard
- 4 or more cloves fresh garlic, shaved or pressed

Add fresh and/or dried herbs:
Add tarragon, basil, oregano, marjoram, garlic powder, or others to taste

Optional additions: 1 can of beans of your choice, green or red onions, pine nuts, diced prunes, dried cranberries, chopped spinach, kale, Swiss chard, or any vegetable of your choice.

Veritable Veggie Nut Loaf

I never think of veggie burgers as a substitute for hamburgers. I just think of them as another kind of food. I feel the same way about nut loaf. Here is a recipe that I developed after a friend made a similar one for Thanksgiving dinner.

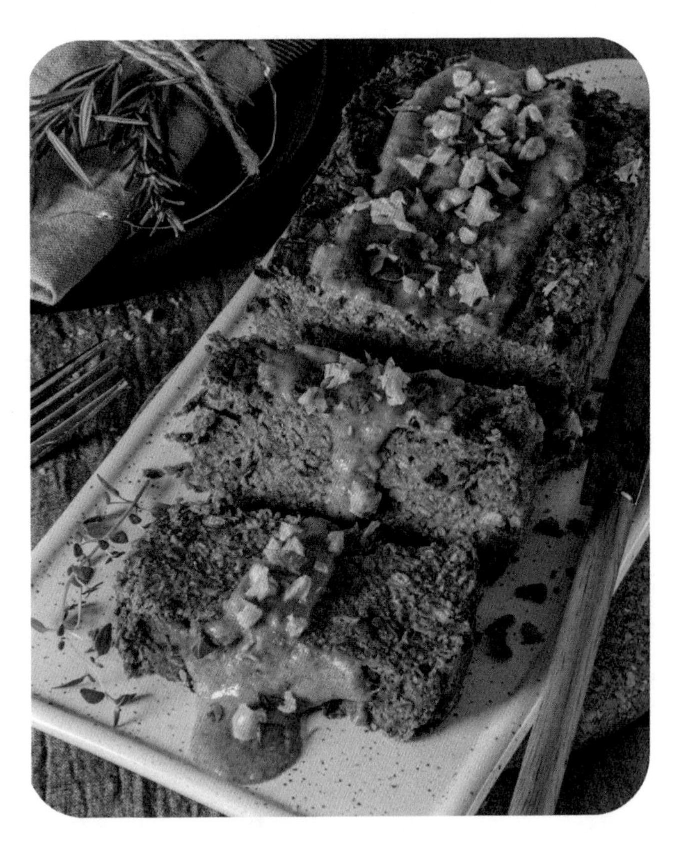

Pre-cook 1 C short grain brown rice in 2 C water (2-to-1). Don't over-cook the rice. You want it slightly nutty in texture. Let cool when done.

While rice is cooking, mince in food processor, blender, or chop finely:

- 1 C almonds
- 1 C walnuts
- 1 C raw cashews
- 1 C raw or roasted peanuts
- 1 large bunch of parsley

Dice & saute:

- 4 large carrots
- 1 large red onion
- 1 large yellow onion

Optional: add 1 large red pepper and 1 large green bell pepper, chopped.

After sauté, add herbs of your choice: marjoram, oregano, basil, tarragon, cumin.

Dice and set aside: 5-6 large celery stalks. Add cooled rice to other ingredients in a large bowl.

ADD: ½ to 1 tsp salt, 4-6 T tamari (soy sauce), some balsamic, some honey, some garlic granules, 2 cloves fresh garlic, ⅓ C olive oil, 6-8 eggs

Mix thoroughly. Bake at 350°F for 45 minutes.

Optional: Add grated cheese during the last 20 minutes of baking.

Gourmet Potatoes "Rotten"

(So named by my daughter at age seven—her favorite dish)

This is a variation on scalloped potatoes but a little richer due to the sour cream. This recipe is easy to make and is a big hit at any event! You might just want to bring a copy of the recipe along with you for friends and family because they will certainly be asking you for it.

Preheat oven to 350°F.

- Pre-cook potatoes - not completely cooked.
- Let potatoes cool and slice in full or half slices.
- (Another option is to grate the potatoes - gives a wonderful taste.)

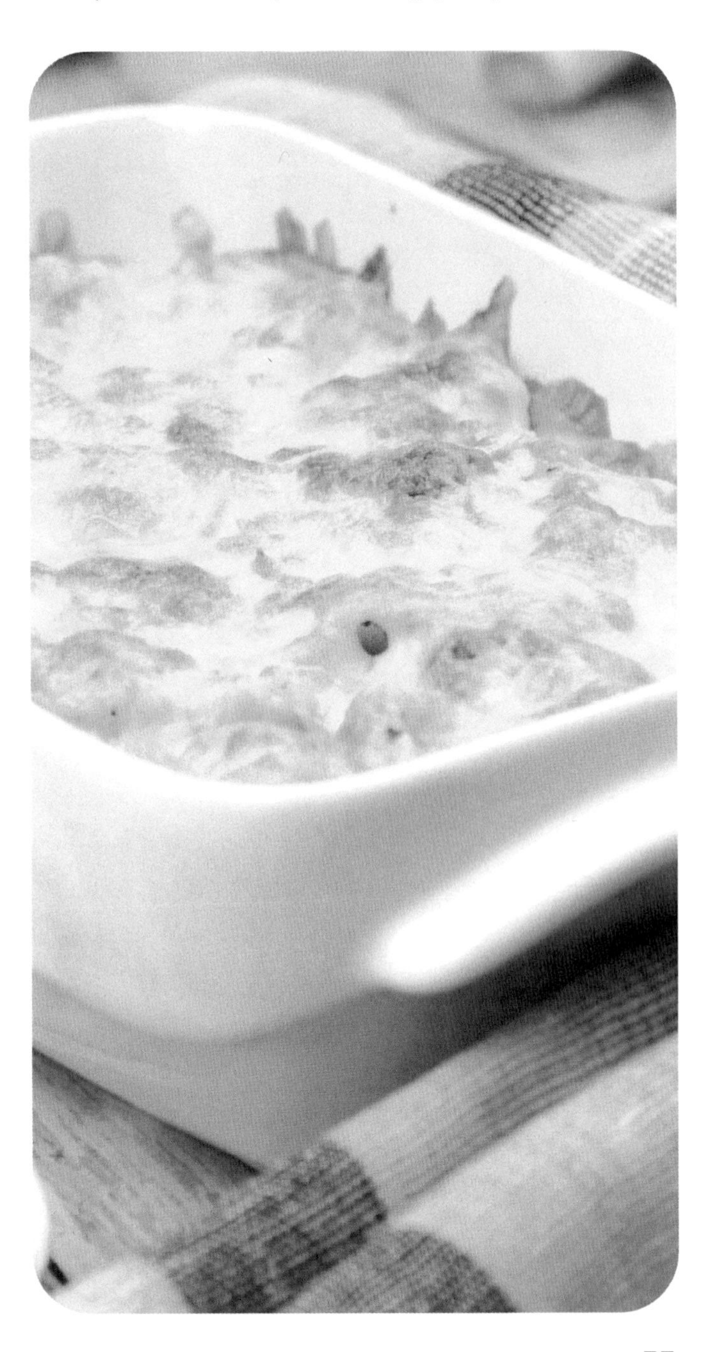

To Prepare:

In casserole dish, make two layers of the following:

- potatoes
- spread with a generous amount of sour cream
- salt
- grated cheese - be generous (Use jack, cheddar and/ or Swiss—a combination is yummy.)

Bake at 350°F for 45 minutes to 1 hour. Cover with foil for the first 30 minutes and then uncover to brown. The browner, the yummier!

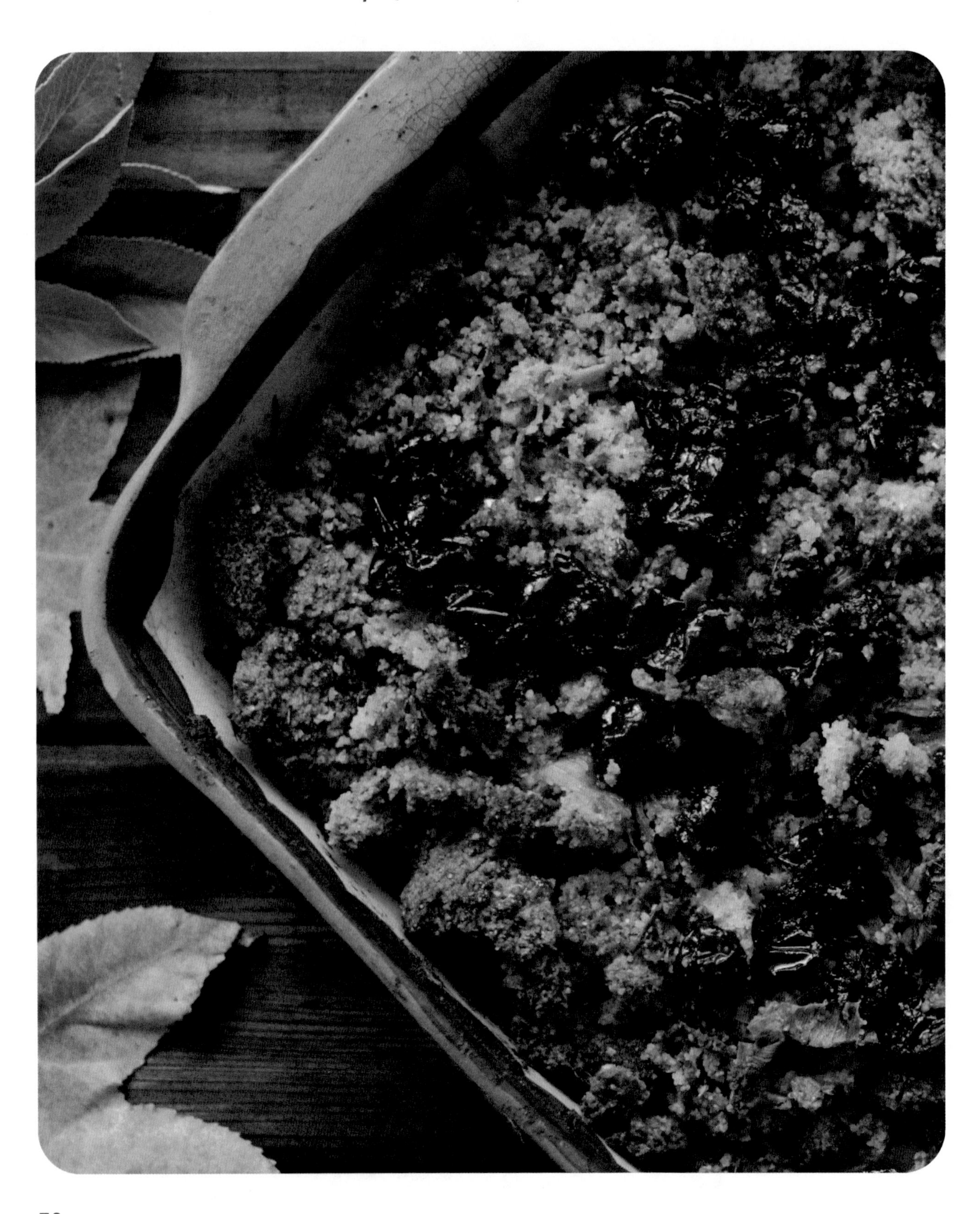

Delicious Cornbread Stuffing

I love cornbread stuffing - most people do. This vegetarian recipe can be made any time of the year. Instead of a turkey, we will be stuffing it into a casserole dish. For Thanksgiving I double this recipe. You can use any cornbread. Included is a delicious cornbread recipe that gives the casserole a special rich flavor.

Make one 8 x 13 inch pan of cornbread. Use your recipe, a boxed mix, or this one.

MOLASSES CORNBREAD

- 3 C cornmeal
- 1 C whole wheat flour
- 4 tsp baking powder
- 1 tsp sea salt
- 1 C honey
- 1 C molasses
- 2 eggs
- 2 ½ C milk
- 1 stick butter or ¼ C olive oil

Bake at 400°F until fork comes out clean.

FOR STUFFING Combine:

- 1 C diced celery
- 1 C diced onion
- 1 stick butter or ¼ C olive oil

Lightly sauté celery and onion in butter or olive oil. (The butter takes the place of broth.) Crumble cornbread in large bowl with sauteed veggies.

Add:

- 4-6 eggs, beaten
- ½ C or more, chopped walnuts
- ½-1 tsp salt to taste
- Herbs: fresh parsley, tarragon, oregano, basil, marjoram, cumin or your choice
- 2 T water
- ½ C light olive oil or butter
- 2 C (more or less) organic corn flakes
- ***Optional:*** 2+ cloves garlic, dried or fresh cranberries, dash of balsamic vinegar

Put into a well-oiled casserole dish and bake at 400°F until fork comes out clean.

Norman's Awesome Cranberries

Every Thanksgiving and Christmas, my father-in-law, Norman, would make these amazing cranberries and taught me. I try to use organic berries, but any will do. Great with any dinner or just to eat by the spoonful. Yum, Yum! Thank you, Norman.

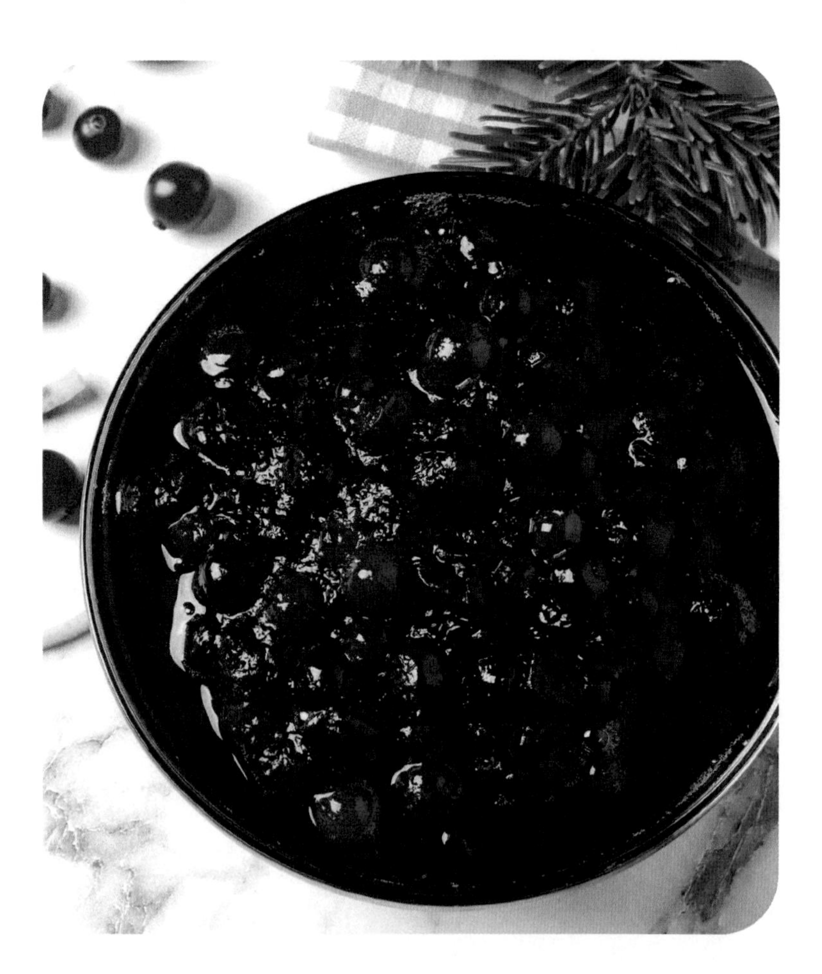

Ingredients:

- cranberries, organic
- sugar, organic
- oranges or mandarins

To Prepare:

Rinse cranberries and remove any damaged ones.

Put the raw, whole cranberries into a saucepan. Use a larger pan to make a bigger batch.

Barely cover with water. Too much water will prevent them from setting.

Add sugar to taste. I use organic sugar. You may have to taste several times to get it right.

Bring to a boil and lower the heat to keep them simmering and bubbling. Stir occasionally and taste after they cook and begin to thicken. When they begin to thicken, turn off the heat and let them sit until cool enough to put into the refrigerator to gel.

Serve in pretty glass dishes to show their amazing color. I usually put 2 or 3 dishes on the Thanksgiving table for easy reach.

Optional: Add pieces of orange or mandarin peel, or pieces of the sliced fruit.

A-Cup A-Cup A-Cup A-Cup Perfect Crisp

My friend, Carolyn, taught me this easy-to-remember recipe. Choose your fruit: peaches, apricots, nectarines, apples, berries (any) and put together this simple yet stunningly delicious cobbler. Often I don't have enough peaches or berries so I fill in with apples. A combination is yummy also. Sometimes I even add diced prunes - incredible!

Ingredients ~ easy to remember:

- 1 C butter, softened
- 1 C sugar
- 1 C whole wheat flour, or any flour (Pamela's Gluten-free is my favorite; it has more flavor.)
- 1 C oats
- 1 tsp salt - don't ever forget the salt!
- fruit (2 C or more)

Cream together the butter, sugar, and salt. Add the flour and oats. I use a potato masher or cream it all together with clean hands.

Spray dish with olive or avocado oil. Put fruit into oiled baking dish and cover with mixture. (Sometimes I put the fruit into the creamed mixture and cover all the pieces evenly.) Bake at 350°F for 45 minutes to 1 hour, or so, until brown.

Always a hit at any potluck or gathering. It feeds a lot of people.

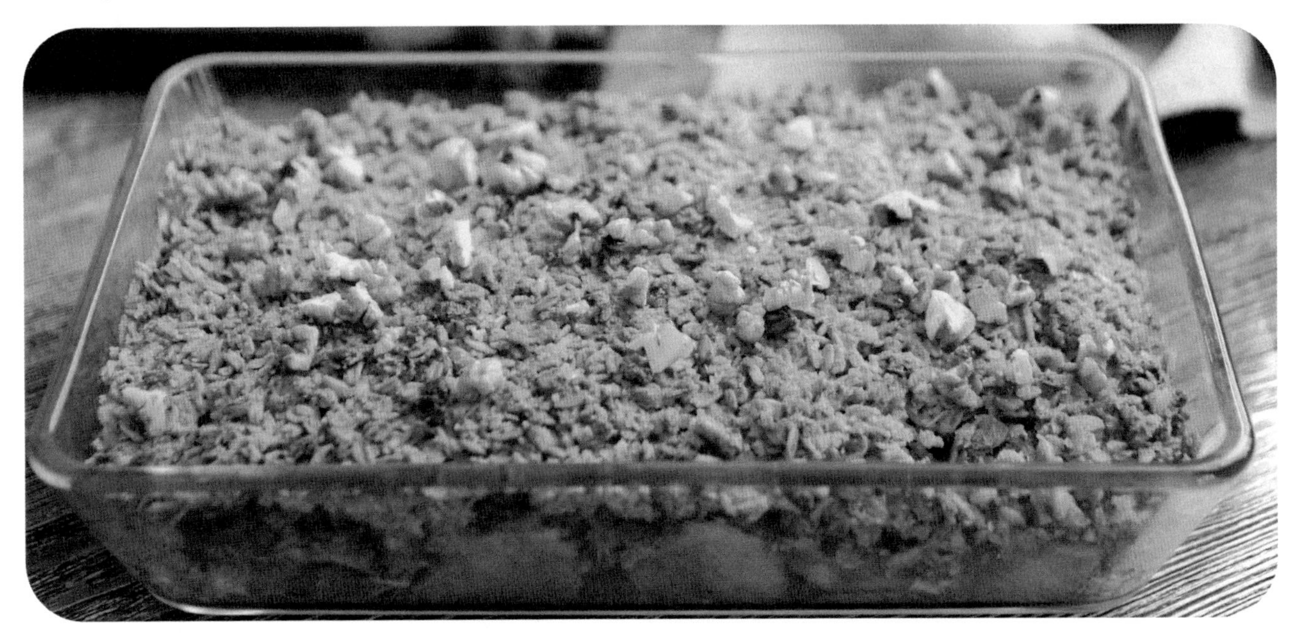

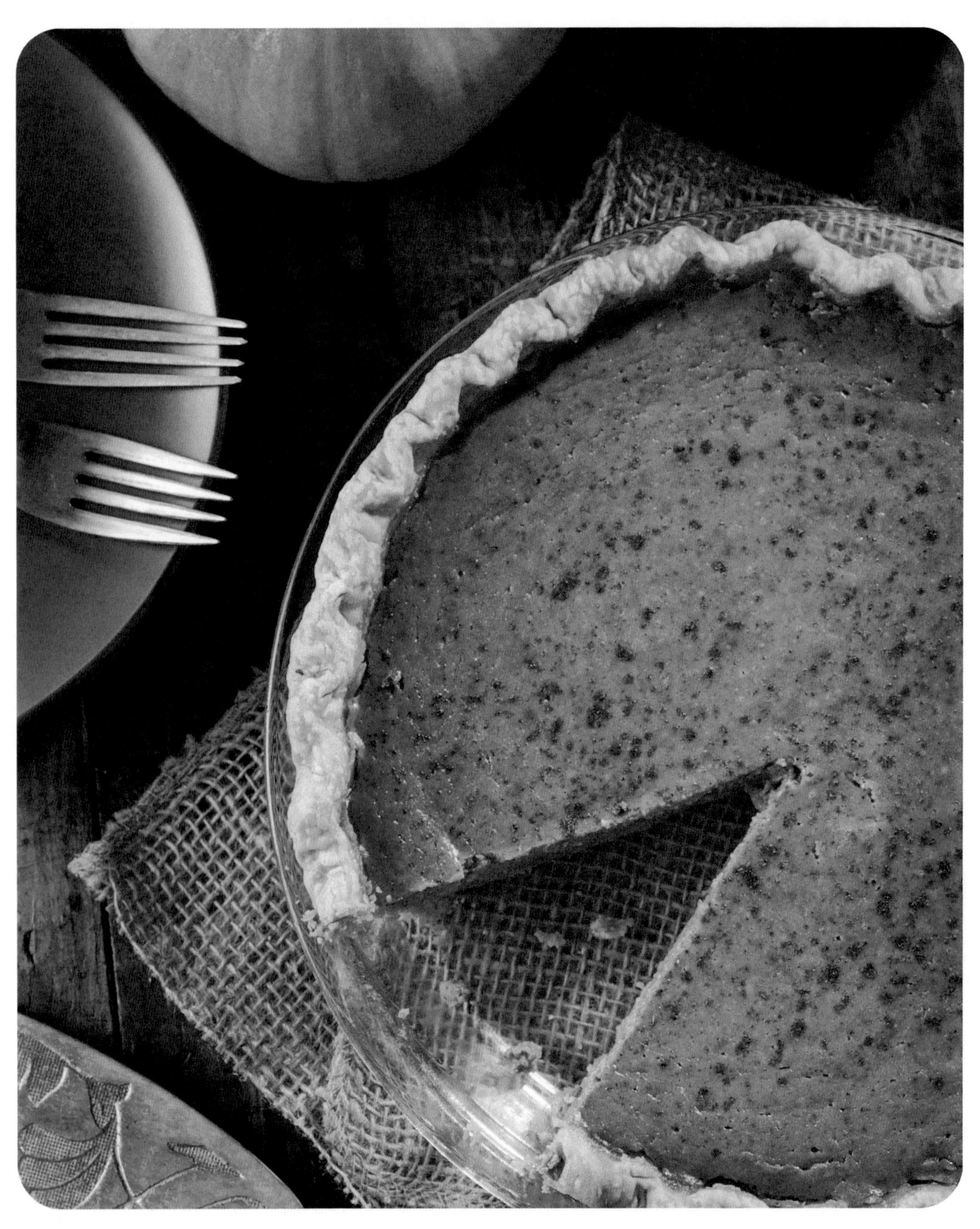

Pumpkin (Not Really) Pie

I use fresh butternut squash instead of pumpkin. Butternut is much more creamy and rich, with more meat. It dances circles around pumpkin and no one can tell the difference. Everyone will be astonished when you tell them you used butternut instead of pumpkin!

Preheat oven to 350°F.

Cut butternut squash into 3-4 inch squares, or bake whole, and boil or steam until soft. DON'T PEEL! Drain water and let cool. When cool scoop out into bowl.

(I cook the squash the day before and put it in the refrigerator. I cook a lot of butternut, about two large ones, and just keep whipping out a couple of pies each day during the holiday season. Once the butternut is cooked, it only takes ten minutes to put the pie in the oven. Baking the butternut gives it more flavor.)

Add to blender:

- 1½ C cooked butternut squash
- 1½ C whole milk, 2%, skim, or soy milk
- 3 or 4 eggs
- 1 tsp sea salt
- 2 T spoons cinnamon
- ⅓ tsp cloves
- 1½ tsp ginger
- About 1 C honey, to taste
  (Remember it needs to taste a little sweeter before it is cooked)

Blend together until smooth. Pour into pie shells. (Yummy with Marie Callender's pre-made shells.)

Bake at 350°F about 1 hour. Makes 2 pies.

This recipe is good with or without whipped cream. When anyone desires whipped cream, I simply put the cream into the blender. Honey can be added, but I don't think it needs it. My Pumpkin (Not Really) Pie is a hit wherever I go.

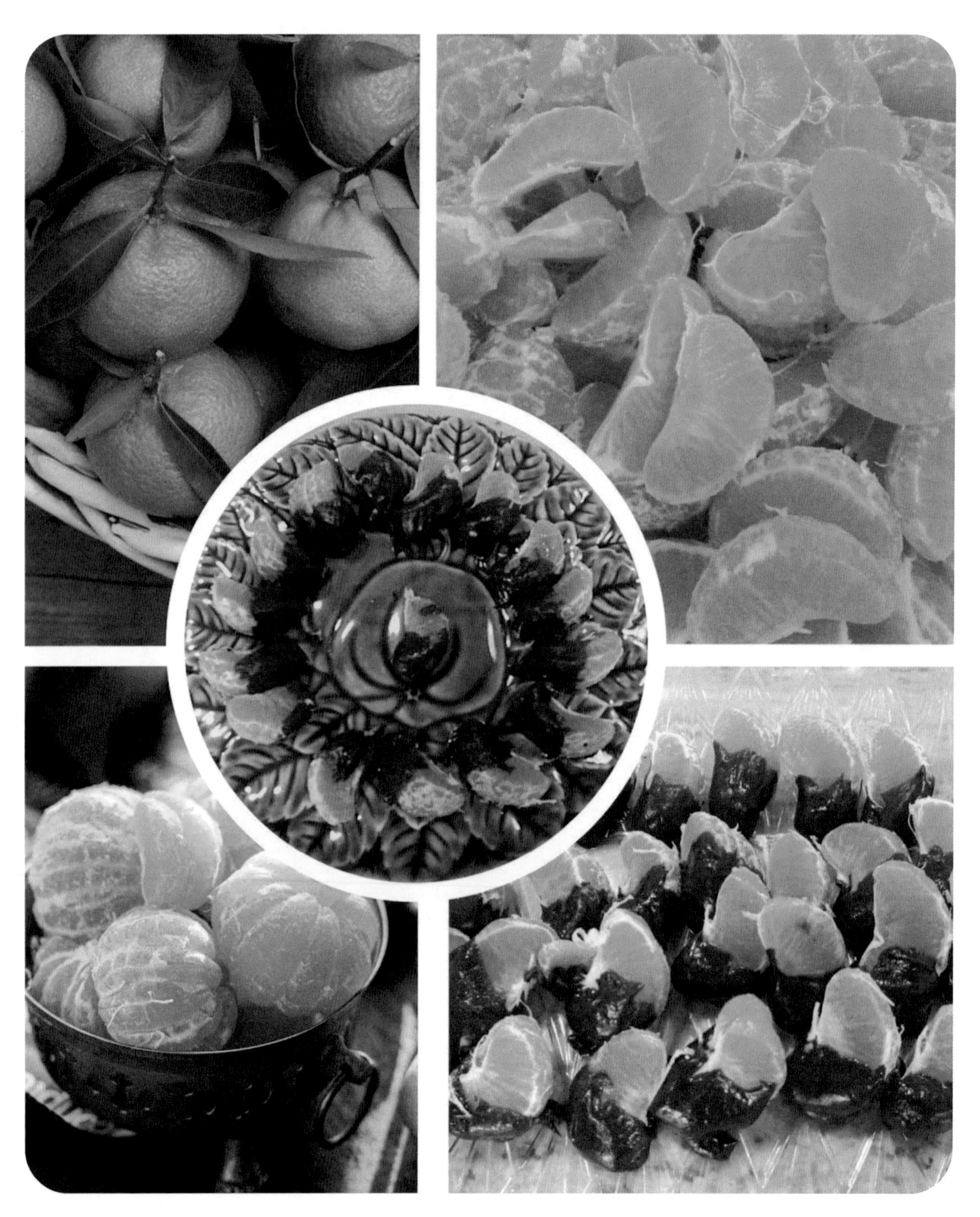

Chocolate Dipped Mandarin Segments

Popular at any gathering - especially Thanksgiving and Christmas parties. For this recipe, I use Satsuma Mandarins that are harvested in November and December. But any citrus can be used. Navel oranges might not work well, as they can get bitter within two hours after they are peeled. Commercial orange juice is made from Valencias.

Ingredients:

- Satsuma Mandarin segments (or other citrus of your choice)
- semi-sweet chocolate chips (or chocolate of your choice)

Use the best quality chocolate you can. I prefer organic, semi-sweet chocolate chips. Put the chocolate in a small saucepan with a little milk and melt it at very low heat, stirring frequently.

Dip each segment half way into the melted chocolate and place on a party tray or plate. I add a layer of parchment paper or waxed paper to prevent the chocolate from sticking. Take to a party and receive tons of compliments.

Ala Satsuma Mandarina

Over our many years of raising mandarins, we have tried many ways of using Satsuma Mandarins. The very best recipe we have ever come up with is as follows. This is the easiest of easy recipes and requires hardly any preparation time.

PEEL A MANDARIN . . . *(The soft ones are the sweetest.)*
EAT IT!

PEEL ANOTHER ONE . . . *(They are so easy to peel.)*
EAT IT!

PEEL ANOTHER ONE . . . *(Children can do this by themselves.)*
EAT IT!

KEEP GOING UNTIL SATISFIED.

Of course, there is another great way to ingest a mandarin . . .
JUICE IT! Freeze it in ice-cube trays!

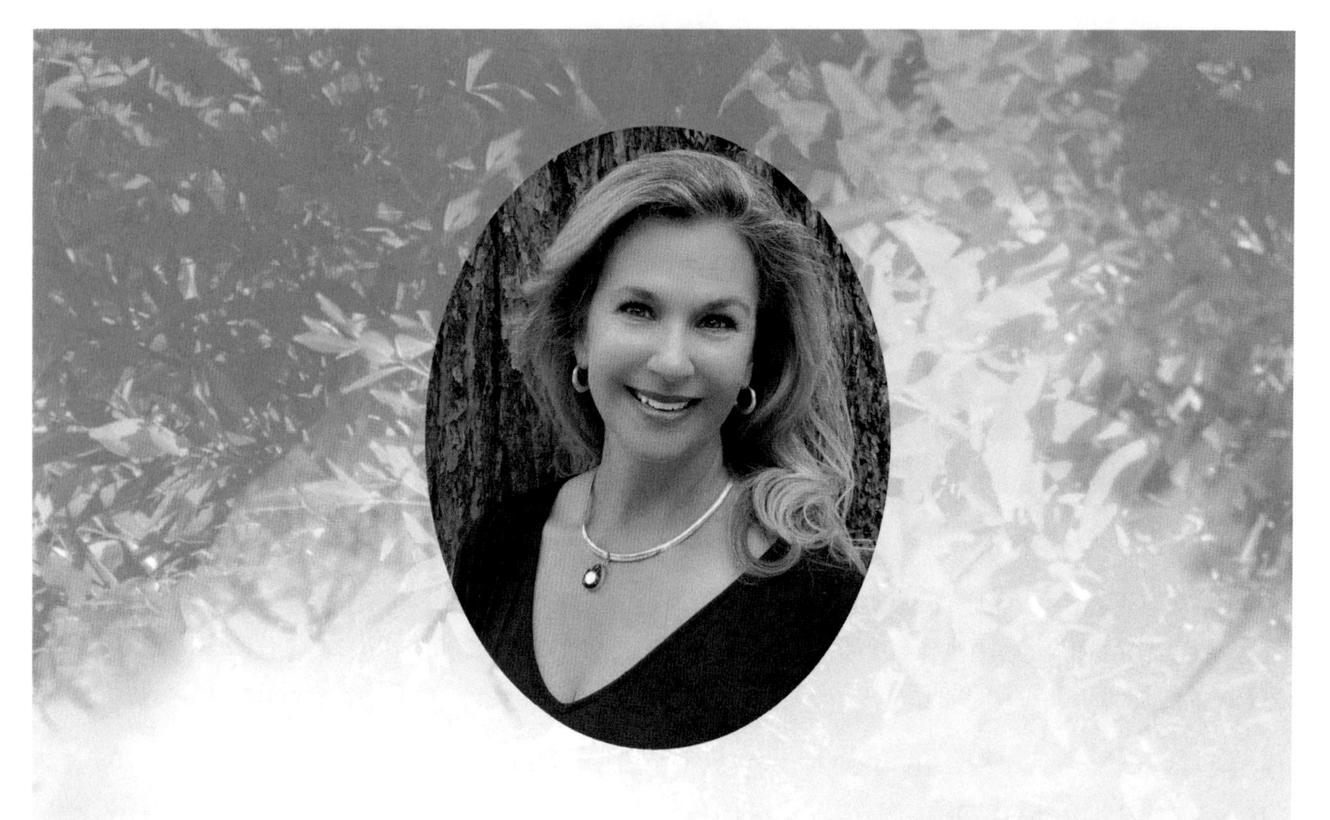

Miriam Lytle

Miriam Lytle is a multi-talented professional with a diverse background in real estate, mortgage lending, and the spa industry. With over 25 years of experience in the real estate industry, Miriam is a licensed Realtor with eXp Realty, working with the Culbertson and Gray group.

Miriam's passion for healthy home cooking was inspired by her Great Grandmother who was born in Sweden. Her love for cooking has led her to create a section in this cookbook where she shares some of her favorite recipes that have been passed down through generations of her family. Two of her Great Grandmother's recipes are included in the book, offering a glimpse into the traditional Swedish cuisine.

Miriam's extensive background in various industries has provided her with a unique perspective on life, and she brings this perspective to her cooking. With her recipes, Miriam hopes to inspire others to embrace healthy eating and explore new flavors, while also celebrating traditional family recipes.

Currently, Miriam is focused on her real estate career, but she continues to pursue her passion for cooking and sharing her knowledge with others.

Email: lytlemiriam@gmail.com

10

Joy Is Found in Family Recipes That Are Tried and True

Miriam Lytle

"Love never fails."

~ 1 Corinthians 13:8

Welcome to Miriam's section of this collaborative recipe book, where we pay homage to the culinary legacy of my beloved Great Grandma Amanda. Hailing from the picturesque landscapes of Sweden, and later settling in the heart of Joliet, Illinois, Amanda was a true Garden Goddess whose culinary creations left an indelible mark on our family's taste buds and hearts.

Amanda's kitchen was a place where magic happened, where the rich traditions of Swedish cuisine melded seamlessly with the flavors of her new American home. Her prowess was legendary, especially when it came to crafting the perfect Swedish pastry crusts and whipping up those fluffy, melt-in-your-mouth Swedish pancakes that have become a cherished family tradition.

In this section, I invite you to embark on a culinary journey through time, tracing the footsteps of my dear Great Grandma Amanda. Her recipes are a testament to her passion, love, and commitment to preserving the flavors of her homeland while embracing the new culinary horizons she encountered in Illinois.

As you explore these recipes you'll see that they are more than just instructions; they are a window into our family's history and a tribute to a remarkable woman who left an enduring legacy through the art of cooking and baking.

I hope that as you recreate these dishes in your own kitchen, you will feel the warmth and love that Amanda poured into each one. May her recipes continue to bring joy, connection, and a taste of Sweden to your family, just as they have for generations in my family. Enjoy the journey, savor the tastes, and cherish the memories.

Great Grandma's Swedish Pancakes

Ingredients:

- 6 eggs
- ¼ C sugar
- 1 tsp salt
- 4 C milk
- 2 C pre-sifted flour
- ½ tsp baking powder

To Prepare:

Beat the eggs, add sugar, salt, baking powder, flour and then milk. Keep mixing throughout the making of the crepe-like pancakes.

Heat a flat, well-buttered crepe pan. Add ¼ C batter to pan, or to desired thick-ness . Flip the pancake when it bubbles and the edges are dry.

Serve hot, with strawberries or other fruit of your choice, plenty of whipping cream, powdered sugar, maple syrup, and even preserves.

Pancakes can be frozen to use later. Makes approximately 10-12 pancakes.

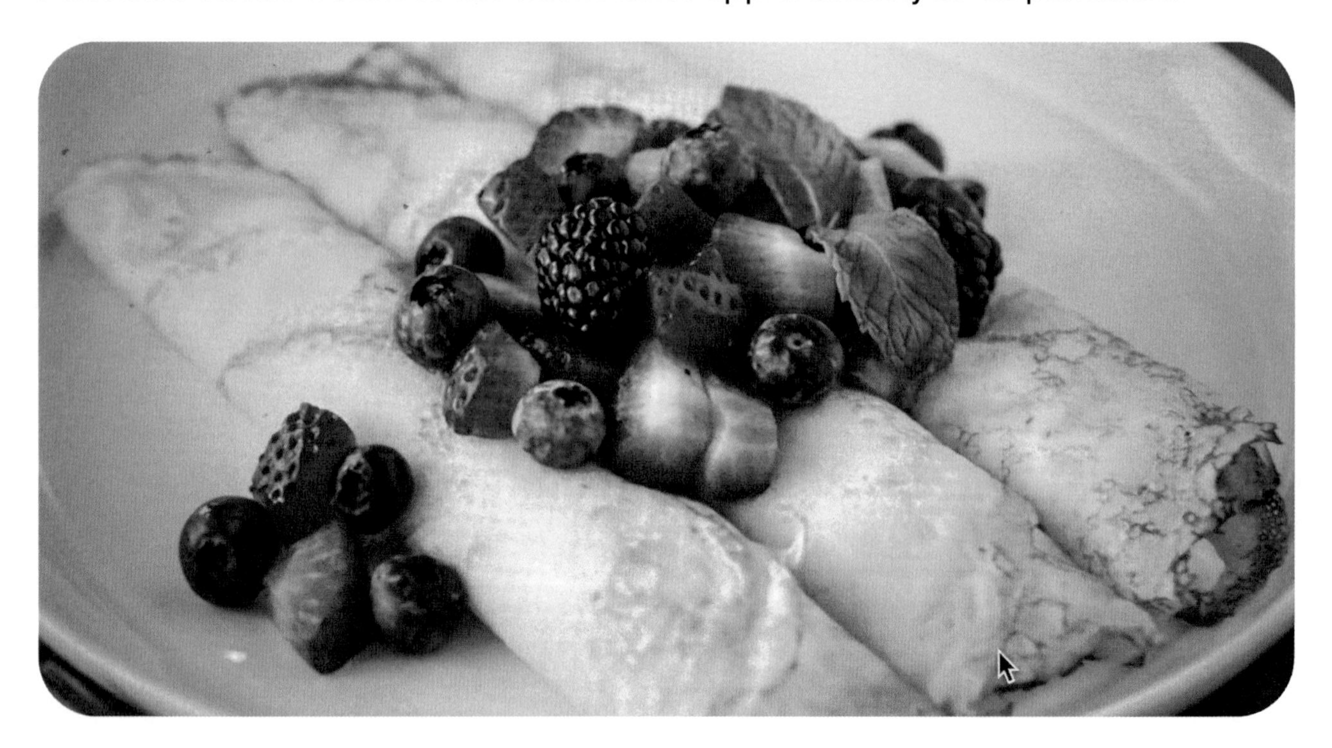

Chili with a Secret Ingredient

Ingredients:

- 1 lb ground beef
- 1 C chopped onion
- ¾ C chopped green peppers
- 5-7 sliced mushrooms
- 1 1-lb. can (14.5 oz) red kidney beans or garbanzo beans
- 1 1-lb. can (14.5 oz) chopped tomatoes with juice
- 1 8 oz can tomato sauce
- 1 tsp salt
- 3½ tsp chili powder
- 1 bay leaf
- 3 cloves garlic, minced
- fresh celery leaves, chopped
- garlic salt, to taste
- sliced black olives (optional)
- 1 tsp sugar
- ½ can beer*

To Prepare:

In a large, heavy saucepan, brown the meat, onion, peppers, and mushrooms. Add the remaining ingredients.

Cover and simmer for 1 hour. Makes 4-6 servings.

**Secret ingredient that helps with the bean side effects.*

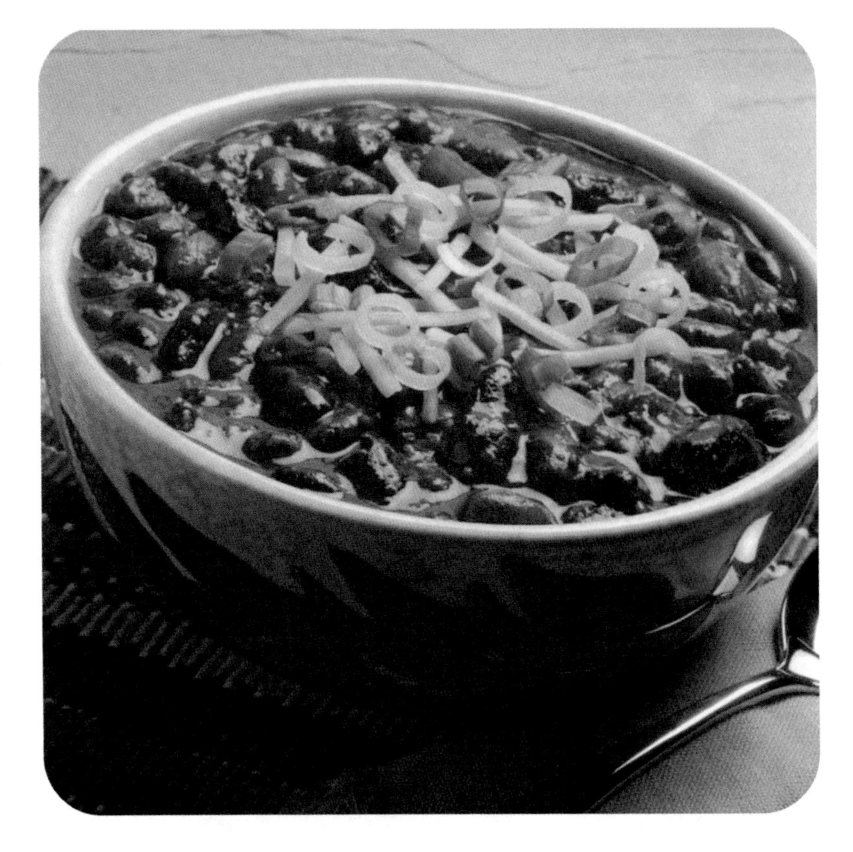

Yummy Split Pea Soup

Ingredients:

- 1 lb. dry green split peas
- 1 meaty ham bone (from holiday leftovers)
- 1½ C chopped onions
- 1 tsp salt
- ½ tsp pepper
- ¼ tsp thyme
- 1 T olive oil
- 1 C diced celery
- 1 C diced carrots
- 2 bay leaves
- 2 C chicken broth
- 2 C water

To Prepare:

Rinse the split peas. In a large pot, sauté the onions in olive oil until clear. Add the broth and water. Add the rest of the ingredients, the split peas, and ham bone. Cook slowly for 1½ hours. Take meat off the ham bone and return to soup. Remove bay leaves before serving. Serves 6-8.

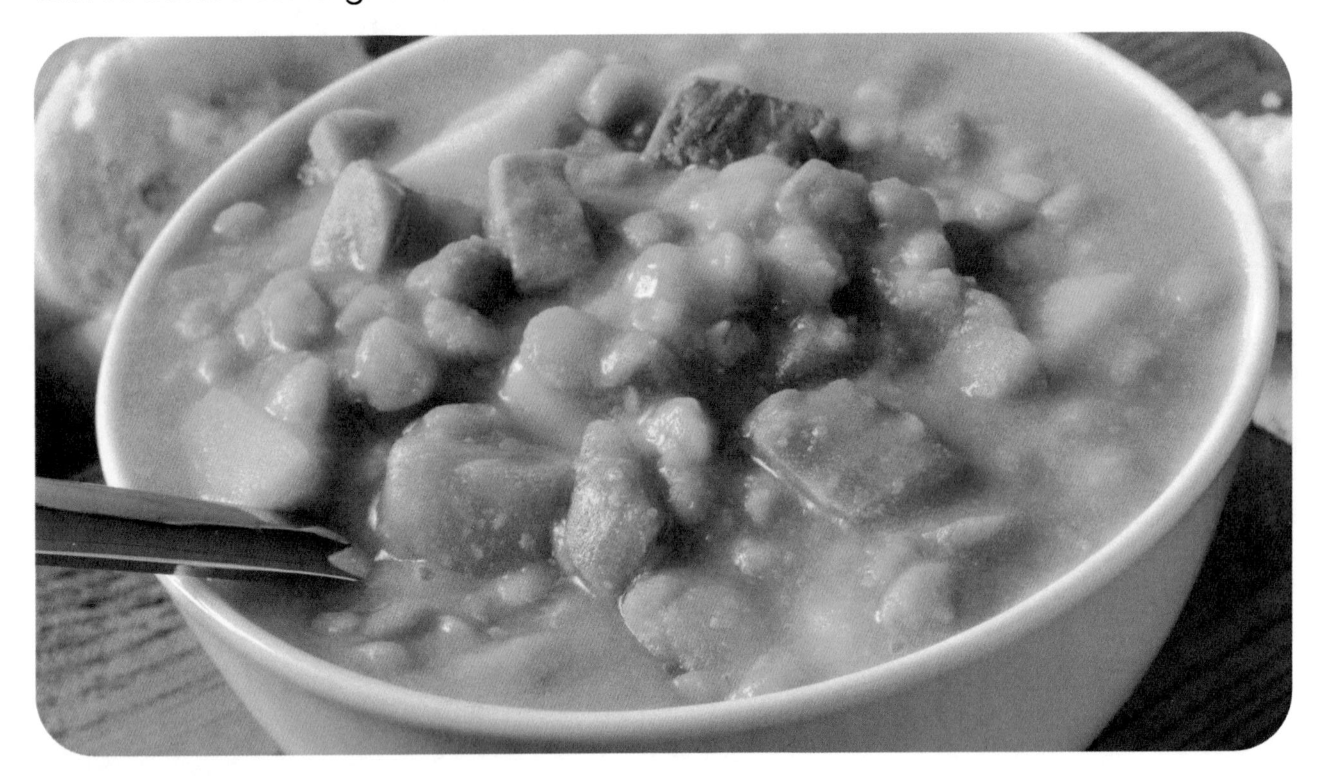

Pumpkin Soup

Ingredients:

- 1 onion, finely chopped
- 3 T butter
- 2 C pumpkin puree
- 1 qt chicken stock of your choice
- ½ tsp ginger
- ¼ tsp nutmeg
- white pepper, dash
- garlic salt, to taste
- salt, to taste
- Wondra flour, to thicken
- 1 pint heavy cream

To Prepare:

In a medium to large pan, sauté onion in butter. Add pumpkin, chicken stock, spices, salt and pepper.

Add Wondra to thicken. Stir in heavy cream.

Heat until hot and creamy.

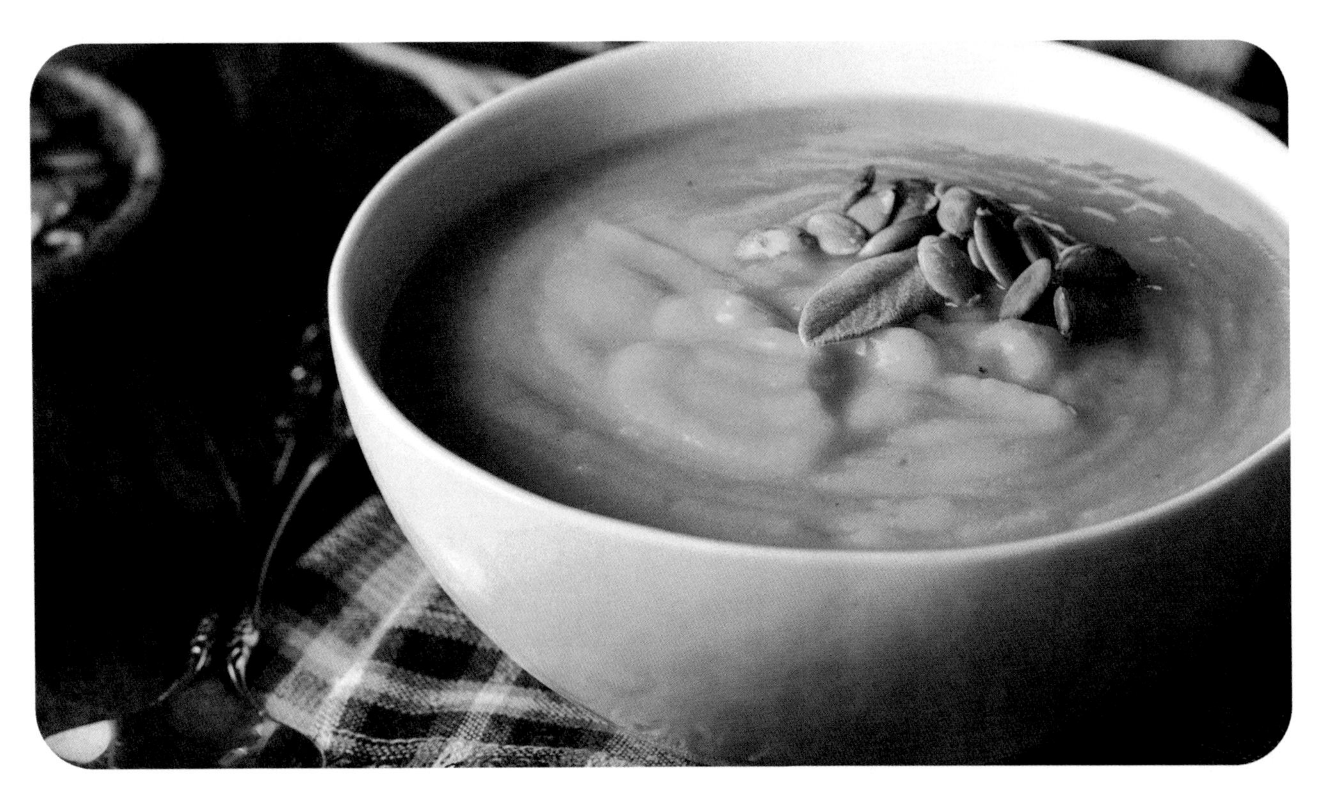

Great Grandma Fredrickson's Pie Crust

Ingredients:

- 1 tsp sugar
- ¼ tsp salt
- ¼ tsp cardamom (secret ingredient)
- ⅓ C butter
- ⅓ C shortening
- 4-5 T cold water (iced water is best)

To Prepare:

Combine dry ingredients. With pastry cutter, cut in the butter and shortening. Mix in the cold water with a fork until all ingredients are moistened and forms a ball.

Separate dough into two balls for top and bottom crusts.

Roll out into rounds and fill with your favorite pie fillings.

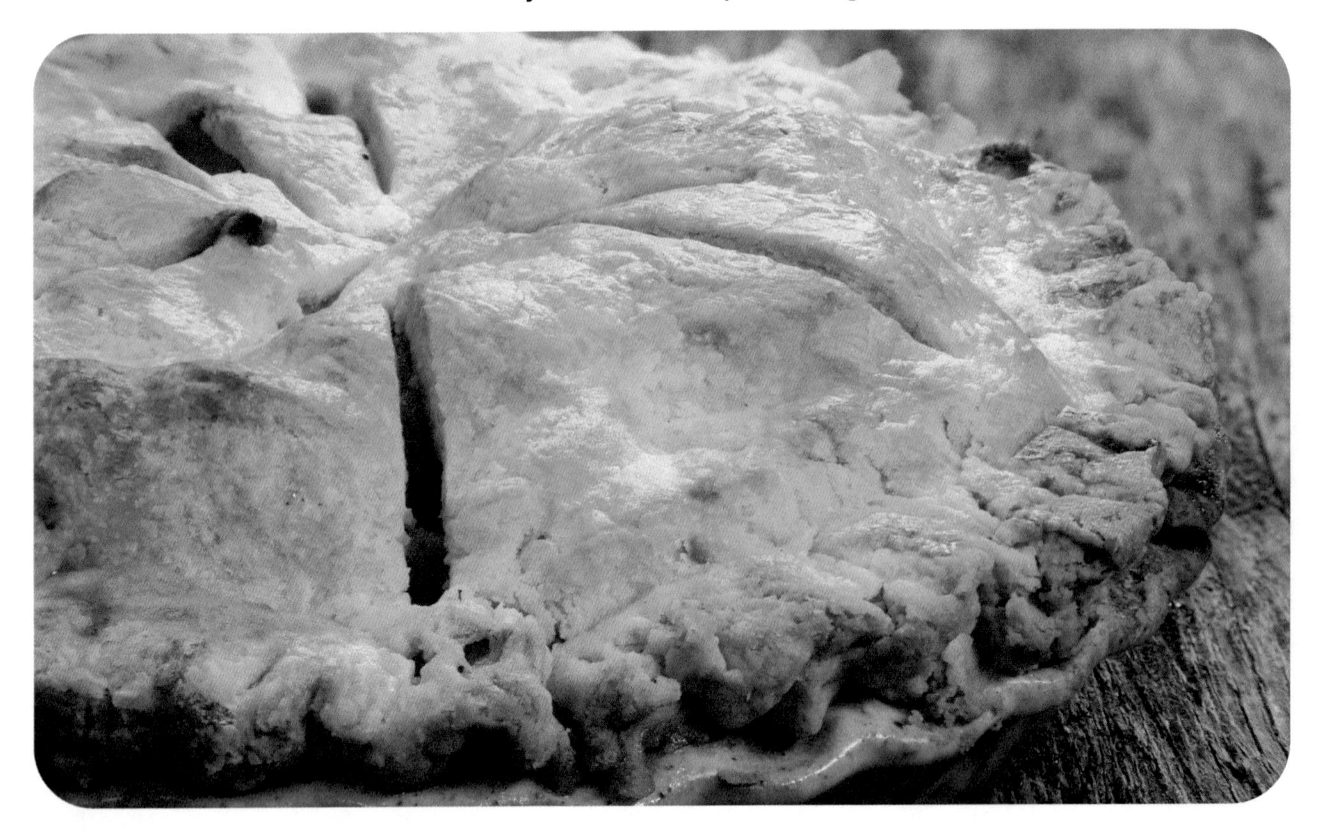

Delicious Dinner Rolls

Ingredients:

- 1 C warm water (not hot)
- 1 tsp sugar
- 1 pkg dry yeast
- ½ C melted butter (warm)
- ½ C sugar
- 3 beaten eggs
- ¾ tsp salt
- 4 C flour

To Prepare:

In a large mixing bowl add 1 tsp sugar to 1 C warm water. Sprinkle the package of dry yeast on top.

Add melted butter, ½ C sugar, beaten eggs, and salt. Add flour, 1 cup at a time, mixing well after each cup is added.

Put the dough into a greased mixing bowl. Cover and refrigerate overnight.

Several hours before serving, cut the dough into two pieces. On a floured board, roll each into a ¼-⅜ inch thick round. Spread each round with softened butter and cut into 12 slices, like a pizza.

Roll each piece up, from wide end to point and place on greased baking sheet. Cover with a towel. Let rise for 3-4 hours, depending on the temperature of the room.

After they have risen and are a nice size, bake at 400°F for 8-10 minutes. Butter the tops while warm. Enjoy! They are delicious and elegant!

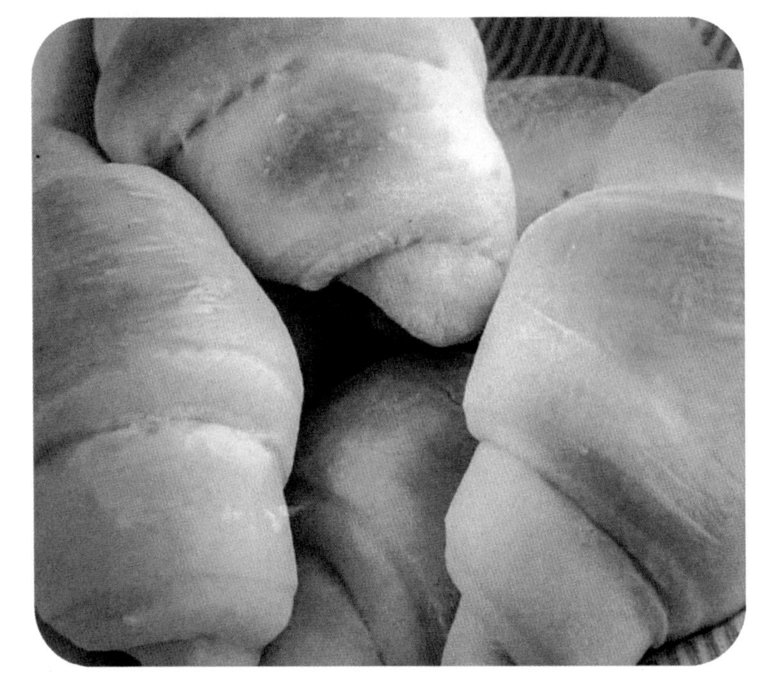

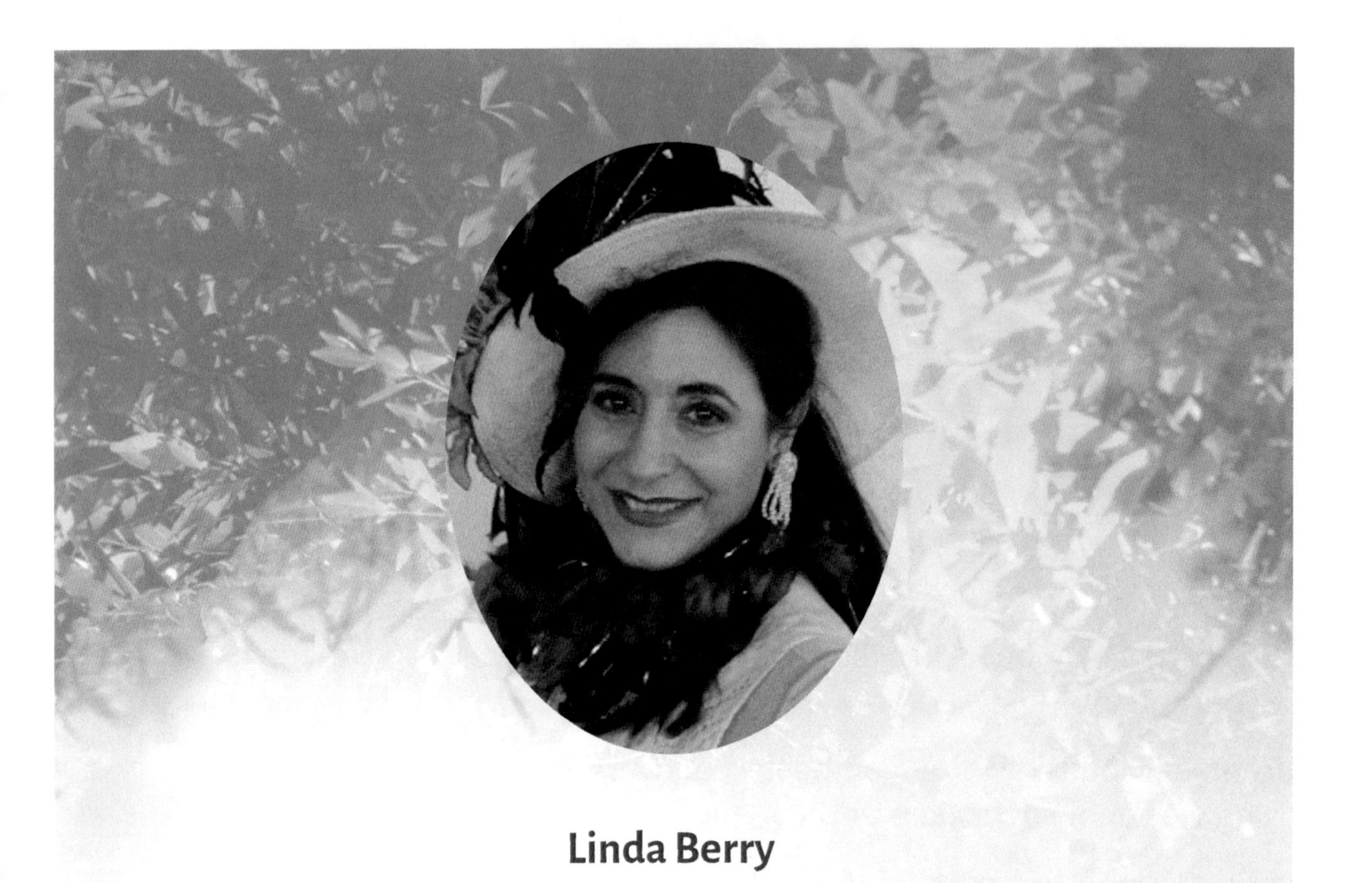

Linda Berry

Linda Berry, founder and owner of BASS (Book Author Support Service) is a multiple bestselling author and professional book marketing and media relations expert. Her books include how-to and self-help, inspirational, children's books, and several series. She owns the Spiritual Discovery™ Center in southern California which offers spiritual, metaphysical, and holistic consultations, courses, workshops, and programs.

Linda graduated from Arizona State University with a degree in broadcast journalism and marketing. She has been a professional writer for over 20 years. Her writings and professional insight have been featured in international publications including *Reader's Digest* and *Woman's Day*. Linda is currently a staff writer and section editor for *Psych News Daily*. She's also a podcast, summit, and conference host, an award-winning presenter and speaker, and has appeared on both radio & television.

Website: www.SpiritualDiscovery.net
Email: LindaBerry_@hotmail.com
Facebook: spiritualdiscoverycenter
Amazon Author: tinyurl.com/LindaBerryAuthorPage
Blog Talk Radio: www.blogtalkradio.com/linda-berry

Tiramisù Italian Cheesecake

Ingredients:

- 6 eggs (6 yolks, 3 whites)
- ¼ C granulated sugar
- ¼ C powdered sugar
- 1 lb. mascarpone cheese
- 1 T vanilla extract
- 6 T espresso coffee powder (dissolved in 1½ C hot water)
- 1½ C of hot water
- 4 T spiced rum (brandy, marsala wine, Kahlua, or coffee liquor may be substituted)
- 1 package of Ladyfingers (24 cookies)
- ½ C cocoa powder
- whipped cream for topping
- grated chocolate for garnish

To Prepare:

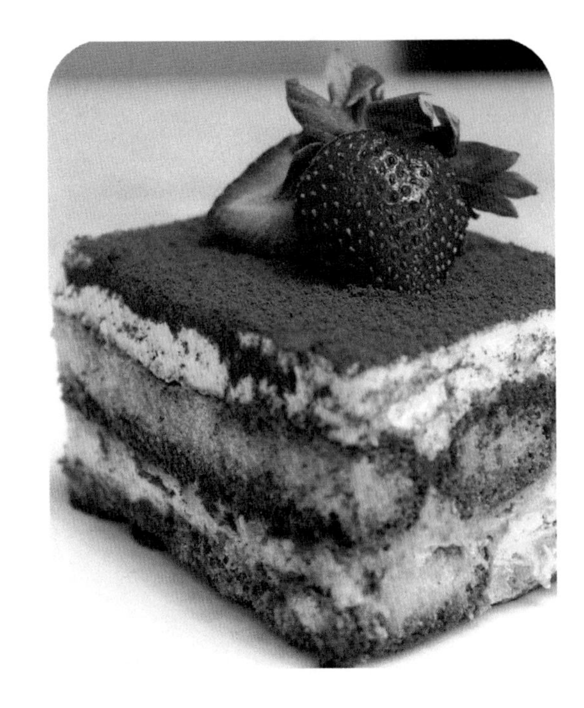

1. In a mixing bowl, whisk together 3 egg whites until stiff peaks form. Set aside.
2. In a separate mixing bowl, use a hand mixer to whisk together 6 egg yolks and the two sugars until thickened and pale yellow, about 5 minutes on a medium-high speed.
3. Add the mascarpone and vanilla to the egg yolk mixture. Whisk until smooth, about 1-2 minutes. The mixture should be smooth and creamy, but not airy like whipped cream.
4. Gently fold in the egg whites. Be careful to maintain their fluffy texture.
5. In a shallow bowl, stir the espresso powder into the hot water. Once dissolved, add the vanilla extract and rum. Quickly dip or brush each ladyfinger with the liquid mixture to wet both sides of the cookie. Do not soak.

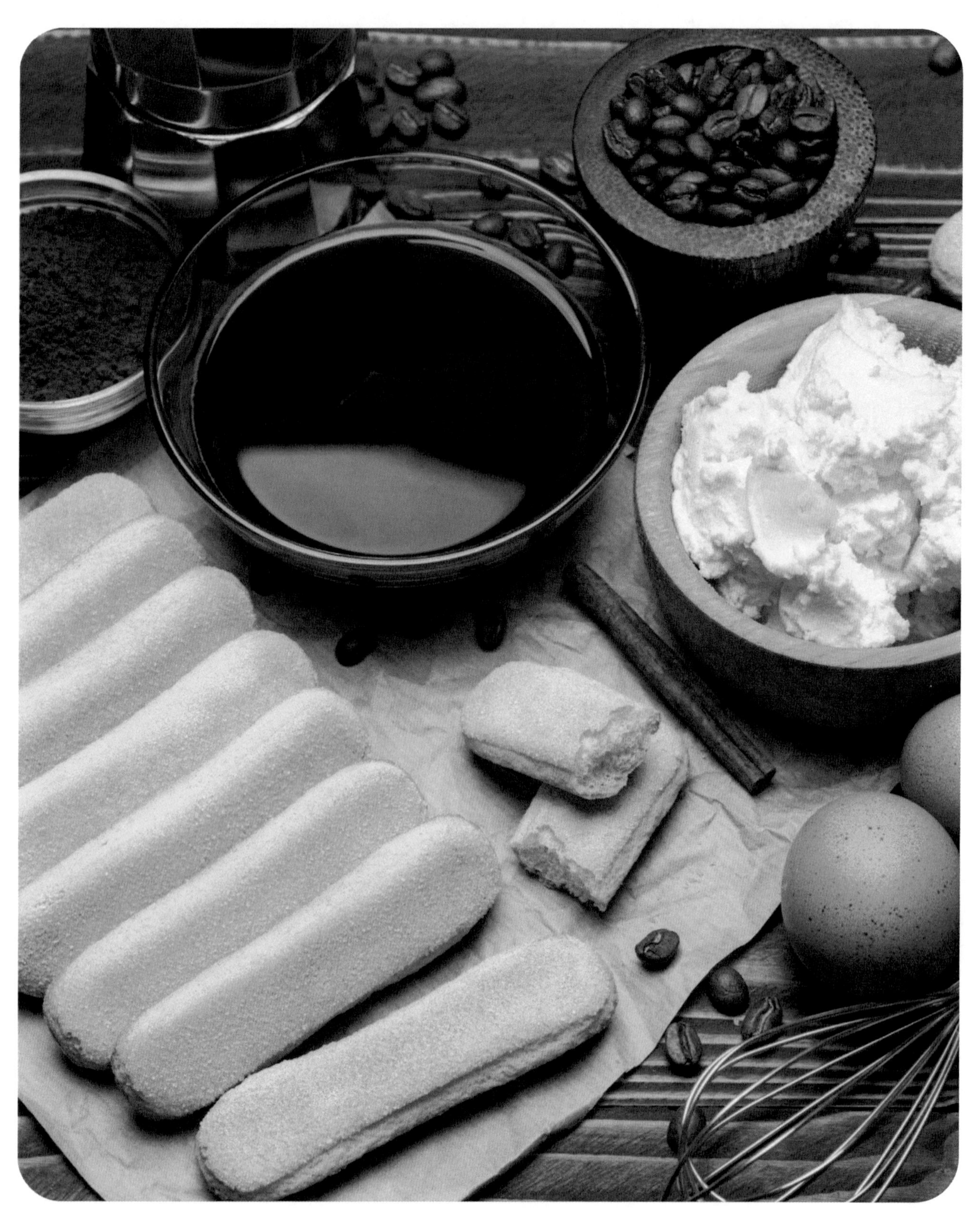

6. To create the dessert, begin with a layer of ladyfingers along the base of an 8 x 8 inch baking dish. The number of ladyfingers needed depends on their size and the baking dish used.
7. Next, evenly spread ⅓ of the mascarpone mixture on top. Sprinkle with ⅓ of the cocoa powder. Repeat the layering of ladyfingers, mascarpone, and cocoa powder twice more.
8. Once finished, cover tightly with plastic wrap. Refrigerate for at least 6 hours before serving.
9. When serving, finish with a layer of whipped cream piped on top and dust with more cocoa powder. Garnish with grated chocolate.

ADDITIONAL NOTES

The dessert name Tiramisù comes from the Italian word tiramisù, meaning "pick me up" or "cheer me up" referring to the two caffeinated ingredients that are in the dish: espresso and cocoa. It's the perfect way to describe this no-bake, rich, and decadent Italian dessert. Records state that Tiramisù originated in Treviso, Italy in the 1800s.

Mascarpone Cheese originates from the region of Lombardy (Northern Italy), mascarpone is a double or triple cream cheese with a spreadable, buttery texture and an out-of-this-world flavor. This rich, sweet and silky-smooth cow's milk cheese is an essential ingredient in Tiramisù. Cream cheese can be used in place of mascarpone, but it's preferred to use the richer, creamier mascarpone cheese.

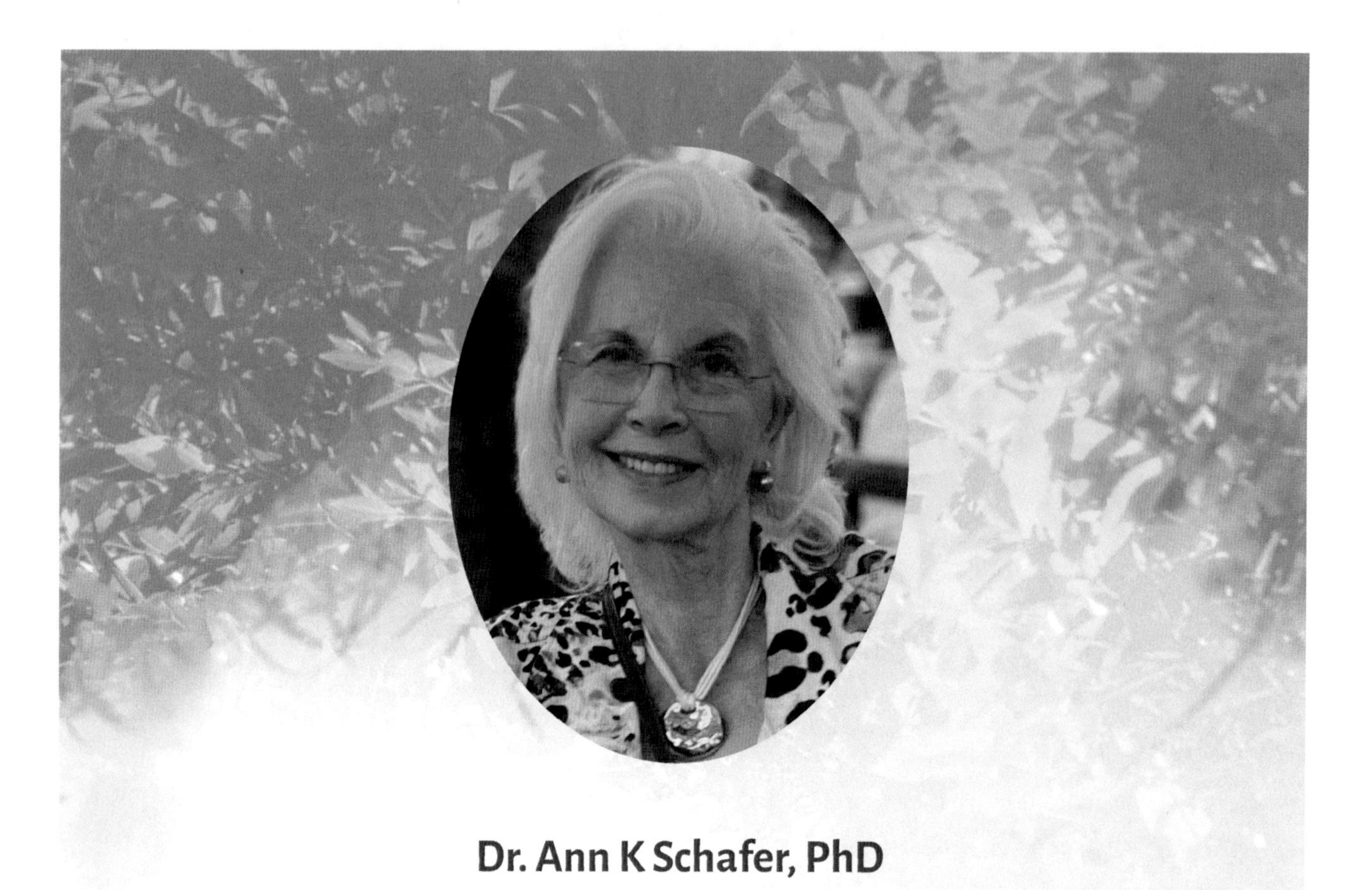

Dr. Ann K Schafer, PhD

Dr. Ann K Schafer is a Professor Emerita at Sacramento City College, a California Community College. She published *Ask Dr Ann . . . About Basic Skills and Learning*, a compilation of her articles from the National Literacy Coalition column, "Ask Dr Ann."

She is a licensed clinical psychologist and holds a certification in Neuropsychology from UC Berkeley. She has worked in three colleges and for seven hospitals. Her current book, *The SoulGrowth Solutions*, examines the healing path to wholeness created by an individual's unmet childhood needs. This bio-psycho-social healing program was originally developed by the Italian physician, Dr Roberto Assagioli, under the name Psychosynthesis.

Websites: askdoctorann.com

12

Ann Schafer's Chapter

Dr. Ann K Schafer, PhD

"Quote goes here"

~ author

I'm a retired professor from Sacramento City College. When I retired I bought a bed and breakfast in Groveland, California, right outside the gates of Yosemite National Park. At first, it was just an inn where people stayed to enjoy all the outdoor activities of the area.

People always asked me, "Where's the breakfast?" And I had to say to them, "Well, this is an inn. We provide beds in rooms, not the breakfast." I finally got so much feedback from my guests that I thought, *what would it take to put breakfast in the mix here?* And so, I got busy with the county and got a license to do it.

The breakfast menu evolved over years of trying all sorts of recipes with eggs, toast, and the basics. But then I began to realize that we were an upscale place in Groveland, on Highway 120 on the way to Yosemite, a very well-traveled road. So I began developing more complex recipes for a more gourmet breakfast offering.

I originally went to Groveland because I bought a 240-acre ranch—if you can believe that! I bought it with my college sweetheart from UC-Davis. He ran the intramural sports program and was a jock. We didn't stay together in college but later got back together and decided we belonged together.

I was coming out of a divorce and had some money to spend, so I bought a ranch. Isn't that what everybody does? No, it's not. And it was crazy. He had gone on to major in farming and ranching at Cal Poly in San Luis Obispo and he knew all about soil and animals. He was also an all-star in every sport, mostly in cycling, and he trained athletes. He was a triathlete at age 51 and became first in California. Number one!

I had some money and he wanted to have a ranch. So I bought the ranch and we had 200 head of sheep and 30 cow/calf pairs. He knew all about it. I didn't, but I knew how to make money. So one thing I learned very quickly: you don't make money very easily unless you have a lot of animals, and we didn't have a lot. 200 head of sheep and 30 cows are not enough to make money.

I saw this inn for sale on Main Street in Groveland and I thought, this could be fun, because I know what to do with hospitality. I had created many events from big conferences to small services. This was an opportunity to utilize my hospitality skills.

The inn was as darling as you could get and had been renovated in 1999. It was built a hundred years earlier in 1899 by one of the prominent townsfolk in Groveland. The woman it was built for had 11 children in it, and later it was renovated and refurbished into an inn.

The Inn was beautifully designed, and all of the rooms are named after places in Yosemite. It features murals painted by Judith Grossman, who is a world class muralist, known all over the United States, and internationally. She painted a mural for each one of the rooms.

Eagles Tower has seven eagles hidden in its mural. You get a prize if you can find all of the eagle heads in the mural. Another mural is named Emerald Pool, which is a place in Yosemite. That one is my favorite, because it is so peaceful and serene. And then there's an incredible mural of Yosemite Falls.

So all of that just spoke to me. It just got into my heart. So I bought the place because we were losing money at the ranch, and I said, "Hmm . . . this is a place I can earn some money." So, I knew I could pay for the ranch with the prospect of the inn, and I did.

I sold the inn during the pandemic. The person who bought it, with a lease option to buy, decided she couldn't make it and so she gave it back to me. So I'm back as an innkeeper and still having fun.

My key to recipes is, first of all, they have to be quick and easy and most importantly, they have to be tasty. The final test of a good recipe for me is, it has to be visually beautiful. So if it passes all those tests: quick and easy, tasty and beautiful, then it goes into my repertoire of the recipes I use and serve. I'll share a few of my favorites here for you to enjoy.

All Seasons Yogurt Parfait

This nourishing parfait can be served for breakfast or keep a few in the fridge for snacks later in the day. It's a favorite here at the All Seasons Grove Bed & Breakfast Inn. People are always very hungry when they wake up, because they're going to Yosemite, or on a rafting trip, hiking, swimming, or other outdoor adventures. We give them a fortifying and delicious breakfast. This yogurt parfait is the first course. I like to serve them in glass ice cream sundae dishes. All of my recipes are quick, easy, and adaptable, like this one.

Ingredients:

- granola of your choice (I prefer gluten-free)
- yogurt (Brown Cow maple or vanilla flavors work well)
- sour cream (the magic ingredient)
- berries, any kind (blueberries, strawberries or a mix)

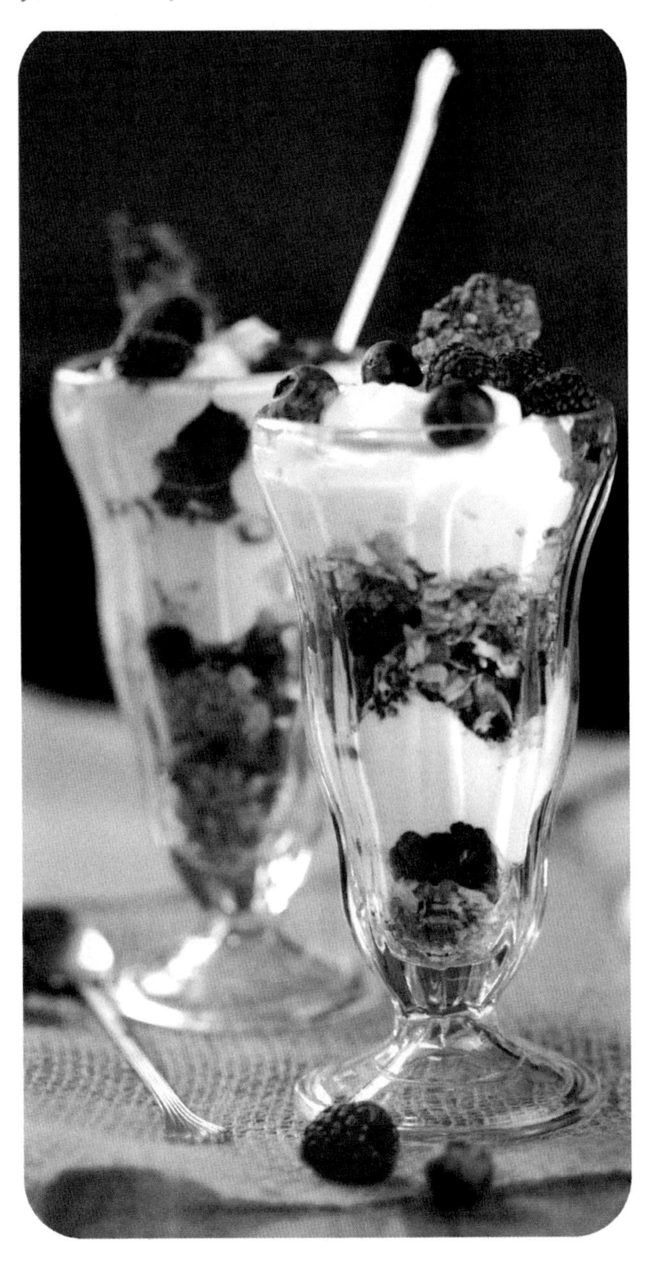

To Prepare:

To make several: mix 2 C yogurt with 1 C sour cream in a small bowl. There are two layers. I like to serve the parfaits in glass ice cream sundae dishes.

First layer:

- 2 large T granola in bottom of serving dish
- 2 large T yogurt mixture
- 2 T berries

Second layer:

- 1 T granola
- 1 T yogurt mixture
- 1 T berries

Last, add a dollop of yogurt mixture with a few berries on top. Voila! Parfait! Yum!

Kitchen Sink Soup

As in "everything's in it but the kitchen sink!" This is an easy potluck soup or quick-to-fix for unexpected guests. It satisfies most palates and is easy to prepare.

To Prepare:

- Start with two boxes of beef, chicken, or vegetable stock in a large pot. (My favorite is miso stock.)
- Add fresh chopped carrots and celery and turn heat to low to medium.
- Add a can of your favorite beans: I like pinto, kidney, or great northern.
- Baby corn is delicious in this soup. Mushrooms (canned or fresh) are good too.
- Add a can of stewed tomatoes or Mexican tomatoes if you like a spicy touch.
- Add 2 T Lawry's garlic salt and pepper to taste.
- Use condiments you like: Worcestershire sauce and Bragg's aminos to taste; I like adding Louisiana hot sauce, rice vinegar, and cumin.

Any meat (ground beef, chicken, ground turkey, pork, lamb) can be added. Cook well and shred to distribute the flavors. Vegetarian is a healthy option too. Certain fresh veggies should be added toward the end, making sure they are not overcooked: (zucchini, spinach, cabbage, etc.)

Great anytime, especially when you need to use up leftovers or are cleaning out the fridge. Be creative and put your own touch on it. Use flavors and ingredients you like. I often add canned or fresh potatoes.

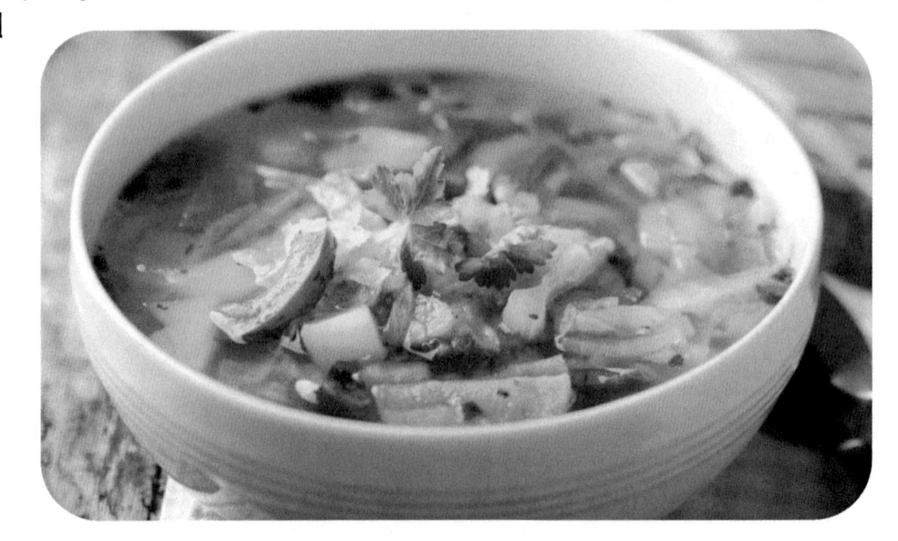

TIP: Keep tasting as you add ingredients. Your tastebuds will help you select what goes well together. This is a quick-to-fix soup satisfies most palates. Create your own version!

Cheery Cherry Cream Cheese Pie

This recipe was from my mother-in-law, discovered early in our relationship when I was a newlywed! To this day, I still can't believe it is so easy and fast to prepare.

To Prepare:

- Bake a premade pie crust of your choice according to directions (don't overbake.) Or use a graham cracker crust pre-made.
- Whip one carton of heavy cream and set aside in the refrigerator. Flavor with 1 tsp vanilla extract, folded into the whipped cream. I sometimes add almond extract to enhance the topping.
- With a hand mixer whip 1 8oz package of cream cheese in a small mixing bowl.
- Next, fold whipping cream into cream cheese with a standard bowl scraper.
- Spoon cream cheese mixture into baked crust and place in refrigerator for at least 15 minutes, or 30 minutes if you have time.
- After cream mixture is cool, take one can of cherry pie filling and carefully ladle the cherry mixture topping on top of cream cheese filling.
- Place entire pie in refrigerator. The longer it sits in the cool fridge, the better it will cut and hold its shape. Even if the mixture is slightly soft, it will still taste wonderful placed in a decorative plate or bowl. A parfait glass is often a good match for this instant goody!

TIP: Try peach or blueberry topping instead of cherry. Change the flavor of the whipped cream, if you prefer. (Try maple, and add pecans to the mixture to vary the recipe.).

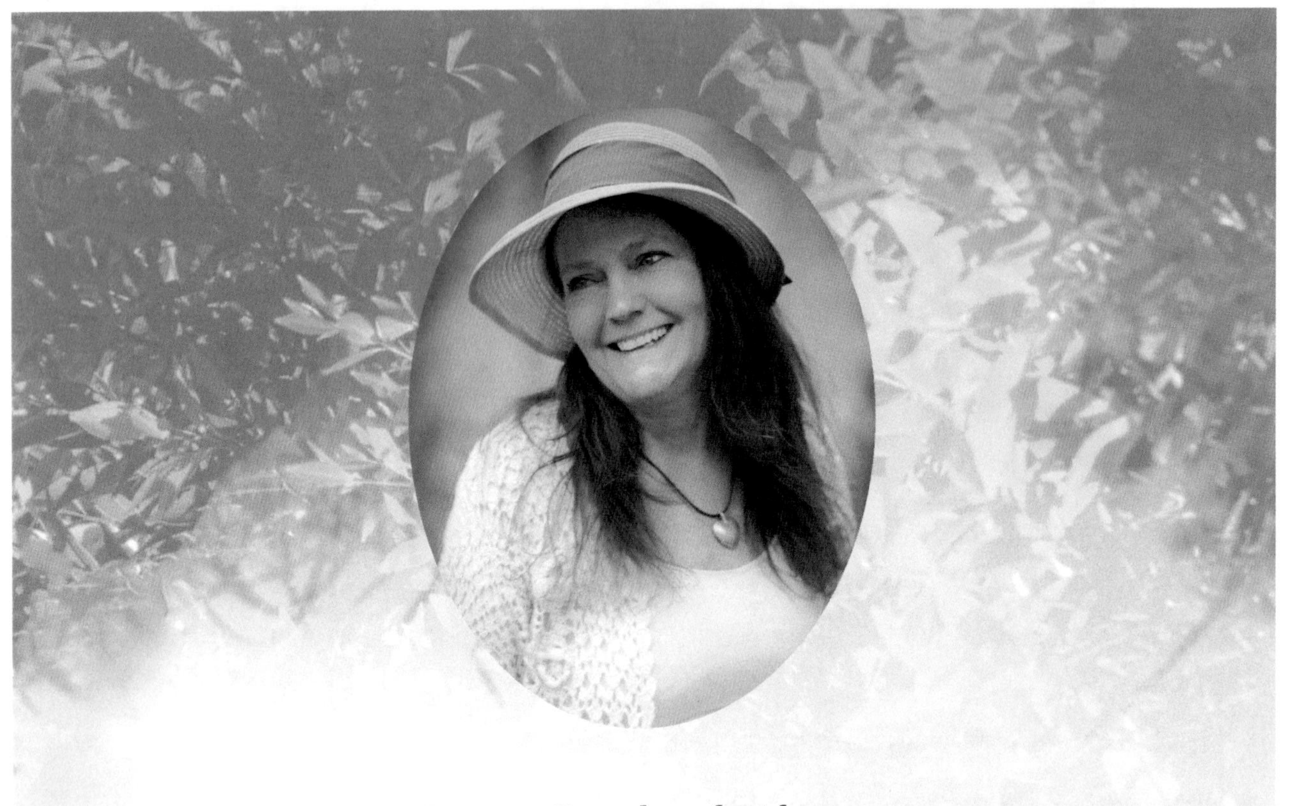

Donna Bosshardt Abreu

As a holistic health and wellness enthusiast, my passion is to educate myself, my family and those around me on how to live healthier, longer and more joyful lives. My passion is to support and coach women towards life transformations of the mind, body, emotion and spirit.

Are you feeling stuck in your life?

Do you desire improved health and wellness?

Do you struggle with speaking your truth or setting healthy boundaries with others?

Do you crave intimate and authentic relationships?

Do you suffer from anxiety, emotional eating or loss?

If you feel exhausted, overtaxed and overwhelmed, my 8-week program is your ticket to stop living your life for everyone else by gaining the confidence to say *No*, with authority and without any guilt or shame.

Websites: WellnessCoachDonna.com
SimplyLivingWellness.com

13

Simply Living Wellness

Donna Bosshardt Abreu

"We are what we eat, breathe, drink and put on our bodies."

~ Donna Bosshardt Abreu

My early days of cooking began as a five-year-old, when my parents bought me a small yellow "kitchen" on wheels. We were living in an old castle in Meggen, Switzerland that had been converted to apartments. We occupied the top apartment, with a round balcony perched on the top of a turret, overlooking the stunning Lake of Lucerne. I'll never forget our kitchen, where my passion for cooking was birthed.

My portable little kitchen had an assortment of small-sized dishware, cutlery and cooking utensils. It came with a miniature hotplate stove that came to a very low temperature, but high enough to feel like a real stove to a five-year-old. I loved cooking in the kitchen on my little stove, alongside my mother who was preparing our family meals.

Fast forward to grade school years, back in the U.S., I still had my little kitchen, but I also enjoyed assisting my mother in the "real" kitchen. My mother would never buy us kids packaged sweets or candy. Yet, I was allowed to bake cookies and cakes to my heart's content, and I quickly learned these talents, as my sweet tooth was rampant.

I remember creating my own recipes for cookies and cakes proportioned to fit my little cooking pans from my portable kitchen. I got quite creative and clever by my making a quick cookie dough recipe that didn't require baking (no mother needed) to satiate my sweets cravings. Pictured below are two of those recipes I found in my mother's recipe box after she passed.

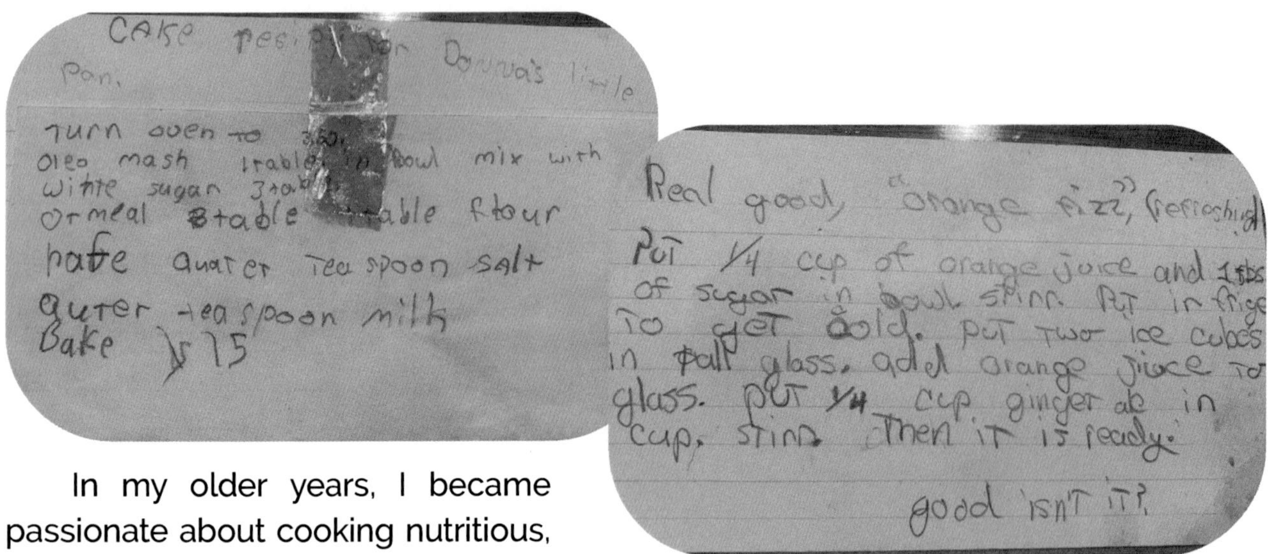

CAke reci... for Donna's little pan.

Turn oven to 350.
oleo mash 1table in bowl mix with
white sugar 3table
ormeal 8table table flour
hafe quater tea spoon salt
quter teaspoon milk
Bake 15

Real good, "orange fizz," (refreshing)
Put 1/4 cup of orange juice and 1tbs of sugar in bowl stirr. Put in frige to get cold. Put two ice cubes in tall glass. add orange juice to glass. Put 1/4 cup ginger ale in cup. stirr Then it is ready.

good isn't it?

In my older years, I became passionate about cooking nutritious, healthy dishes, especially from the garden. I added sprouting, juicing, and fermenting to my repertoire. My favorite baking became flourless, low sugar, dark chocolate nut tortes piled high with edible flowers.

My cooking enjoyment continued to grow. I was inspired by hanging out with the Garden Goddesses, cooking and barbequing with my husband Mike and the kids, and attending large family dinner gatherings. I especially enjoy cooking with my sister, Heidi, who inspires me greatly with her unique self-created, and delicious recipes.

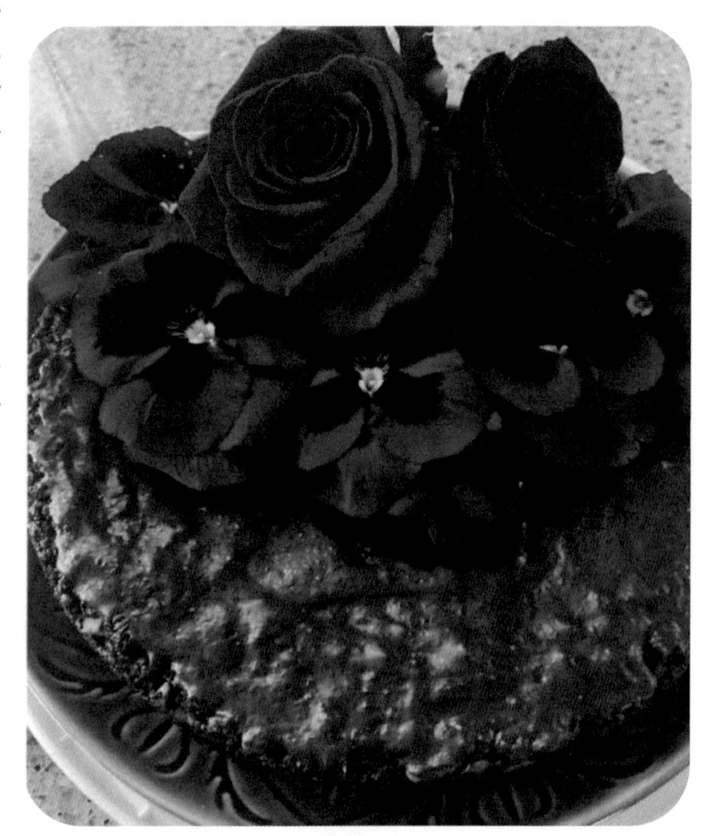

As my life and diet started to make a transition, I incorporated more and more holistic health practices. For several years, I removed cow-based dairy, gluten, soy, and corn, due to food intolerances that I discovered through applied kinesiology. My body would weaken from ingesting these foods. To this day, I rarely consume soy in any form, and avoid corn and gluten as much as possible. For dairy, I stick to sheep or goat, and raw, when possible.

Coconut has been a major staple in my diet. Coconut yogurt is a wonderful treat and a nice alternative to cow dairy. This year (2023) I have been learning about plant toxins including oxalates, lectins, and phytic acid which exist in plants to ward off consumption by animal predators.

Alongside of my cooking and wellness journey, I embarked on a spiritual awakening journey. I am thankful for the many friends, teachers and guides I have met and worked with along the way, including my sister-in-law, Therese. I realize now that everything consists of energy, including foods, rocks, trees, and especially us humans.

I have learned from the ancient Indian medical system, known as Ayurveda, that how we prepare our food matters. If we slave over our stove in a rush, stressed out and resentful of having this chore of cooking for our family, for example, all that negative energy enters the food and is fed directly to our most sacred loved ones! Just one reason the practice of blessing and showing gratitude for our meals before consuming is so important.

I am a different person than I was 20 years ago, and even five years ago: more aware, more conscious, and more connected. That connectedness brings so much more joy and purpose to my life. I finally feel like I know myself on a deeper level, on any level for that matter! I know what I like and what makes my heart sing. I know what I don't like. I know that I have a purpose for being here and chose to be here in this lifetime, as hard as it can seem sometimes.

I finally have an understanding of spirituality, at least what it means to me. It's all tied in together, hence the term "holistic health and wellness." This understanding also began to transform my life. To me, spirituality is going within, connecting with our inner self, which is our spirit.

Spirituality is realizing there is something greater outside of us that everyone is part of. You may choose to call that God, or you may call it Universe, The Great One, Spirit, Source, Universal Energy, Greater Self, Inner Wisdom, or anything else. I like to call it Inner Wisdom. I believe being spiritual is making an effort each day to connect to others, to connect to that inner wisdom, and to connect to Source.

I am still on my journey, and always will be, but I have sense of peace, knowing, and understanding that I lacked before. I understand that wellness involves the entire picture, not just the physical body; it encompasses what we put into our mouths, and the mind body. It involves the emotional body, and especially, it involves our spirit.

If you are interested in learning more about these holistic health and wellness topics, you may join me over at SimplyLivingWellness.com. I look forward to connecting with you!

Cold & Flu Remedies

Healing Socks to Eliminate A Stuffy Nose

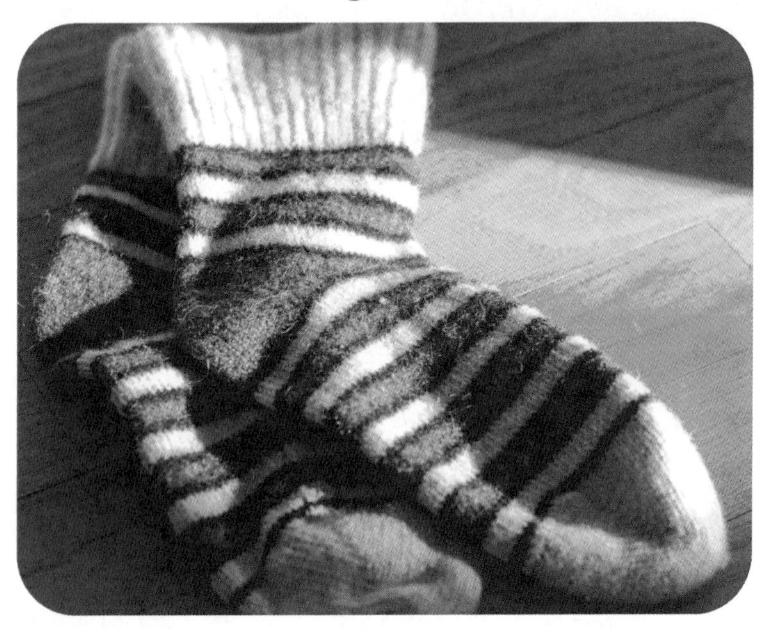

Have bad congestion from a cold? Healing socks work like a charm to clear your nasal passages from a bad cold. After 1-3 treatments, your congestion will be gone. Healing socks induce hydrotherapy, which stimulates the body to reflexively increase blood circulation.

The process also slightly raises your body temperature and flushes your lymphatic system. A well-functioning lymphatic system is important for killing off bad bacteria and viruses, because the lymphatic system carries all our white blood cells around the body. The bad bacteria and viruses that make us sick can only live at normal body temperature, so even a half of a degree elevation will kill them and shorten the duration of the illness.

You will wear the healing socks overnight while sleeping. Right before you go to bed, follow these steps:

1. Run a pair of short cotton socks under very cold tap water. Once they are drenched, ring out the excess water. Have these cold wet socks ready to go.
2. Fill a plastic tub with hot water a little over ankle deep. Make the water as hot as you can bear for soaking your feet. Medium-sized storage boxes work great for this. Soak your feet in the hot water for about 5-10 minutes until your feet are nice and red and hot.
3. Remove feet from the hot water and immediately put the cold wet socks on your feet. Optionally, you may rub peppermint and/or eucalyptus essential oil on the bottom of your feet, then cover with castor oil.

4. Place a pair of wool socks over the cotton socks. These keep the moisture inside as opposed to getting your sheets wet.
5. Immediately go to bed. Avoid walking around before going to bed.

Upon rising, the drenched cotton socks will be bone dry. You have just absorbed all that liquid into your body!

Repeat the next night if needed and a third night if still not clear of congestion. Your cold won't be completely gone; however, you should be able to breathe free and clear through your nose after treatment(s).

> **TIP:** When I have really bad congestion and wake up in the middle of the night, I'll repeat the steps if my cotton socks are already dry. This speeds up the process.

No-Fail Supplements to Kick that Cold

Suffering from a cold or flu? Better yet, on the verge of coming down with something? Try these supplements. There are many vitamins, minerals and herb supplements that help combat colds and flu. Believe me, I have tried them all! I have found the following to be most effective. When I feel like I might be getting sick, I will start this regiment straight away. This routine, coupled with a day or two of rest, usually allows me to avoid getting sick.

Before we get into the protocols, let's talk about the quality of supplements for a minute. Most supplements, even so-called high-quality ones, have added fillers that are not good for us. Even high-quality brands often contain vitamin E tocopherols or alpha tocopherols, which are usually soy-based. Ascorbate acid, citric acid, citrate, dextrose, and maltodextrin are usually corn-based.

Zinc with Quinine

I take 40 mg of zinc daily for flu and cold prevention among other health benefits. I take a 20 mg pill twice a day with food. It's important to take zinc with food as it can make you feel very nauseous on an empty stomach.

If I feel like I am coming down with a cold or flu, I will immediately double my zinc. The magic here is taking zinc with quinine, because the quinine increases absorption of the zinc. I used to use bottled tonic water, but I prefer not to drink the added sweeteners. I now purchase liquid quinine extract and place one dropper full in a small amount of water and drink with the zinc.

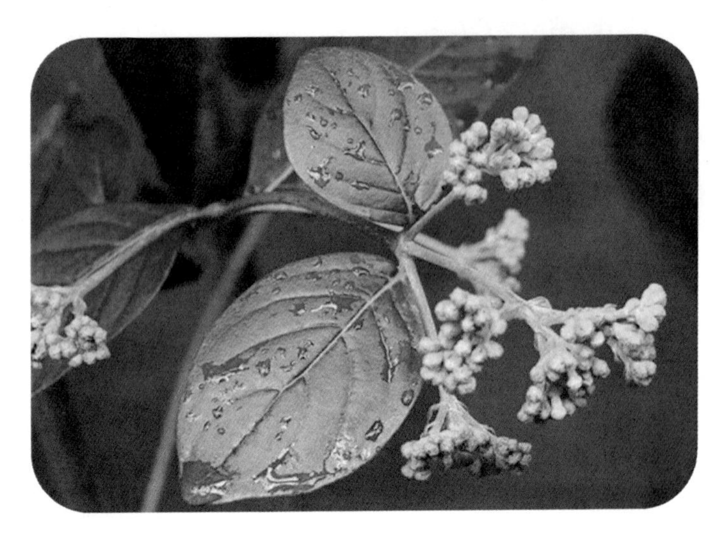

Quinine comes from the bark of the Andean Fever Tree, which has remarkable healing properties which were discovered in the 17th century. These include fever reduction, assisting with digestion, and easing leg cramps. Quinine can also be used to treat malaria, caused by the plasmodium falciparum parasite. You can find quinine extract on Amazon, or perhaps at a health food store.

Vitamin D

Vitamin D is the mother of all supplements. Recently discovered healing properties include reducing inflammation, heart and respiratory diseases, preventing cancer, and extending lifespan.

Vitamin D is best taken as a preventative. If you do get sick, then increase the quantity for a few days. I take 5,000 IU of vitamin D, approximately 6 days per week in the winter and about 5,000 IU on 3-5 days per week in the summer.

Each person's body is different. It's best to take a vitamin D blood test to know if you are deficient; 60-80 mg/ml is ideal. After supplementation, test again to determine optimal dosage. A summer test will differ greatly from a winter test, so frequent testing the first year is important.

Hydroxychloroquine (HCQ)

HCQ is an effective remedy for treat ing and preventing viruses. You can purchase HCQ supplements, but you can easily make HCQ in your home by simmering the skins of lemons and grapefruits in water for two hours.

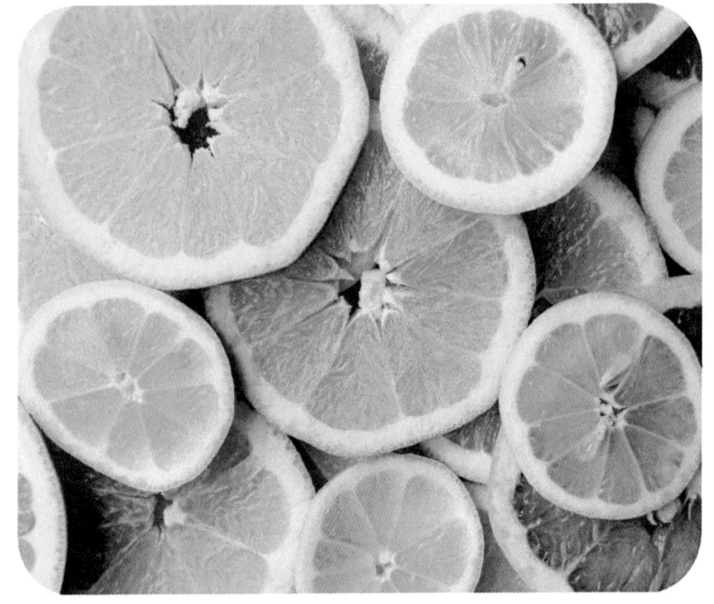

Drain the HCQ water from your pot, then add fresh water to reuse the skins. This process may be repeated until the skins start to break down.

Store the HCQ in jars in your refrigerator for up to several weeks.

Take one shot glass full daily as a preventative, and three times per day when you are feeling sick.

Homemade Chicken Broth

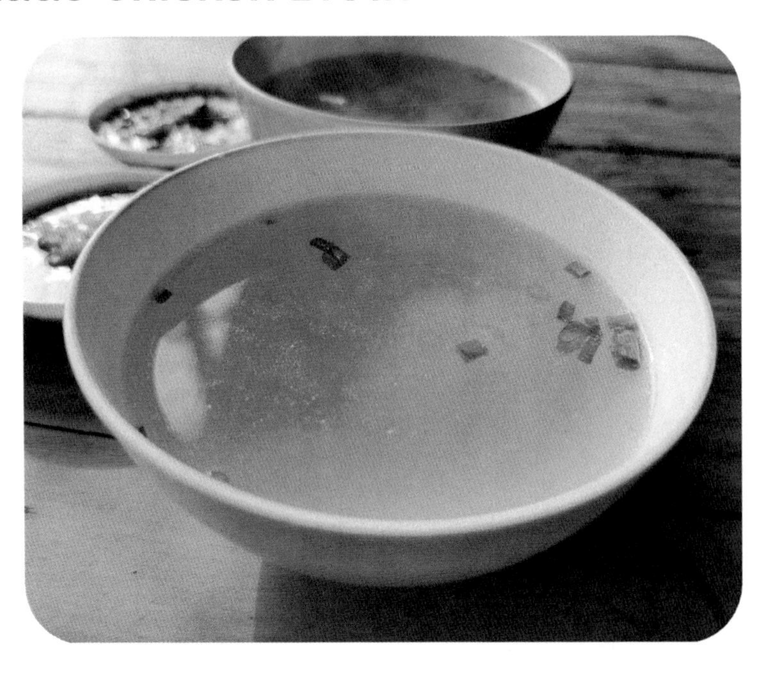

Bone broth is sometimes referred to as "Jewish penicillin" because the Jewish people have long used bone broth to promote healing in the body. I love the taste of chicken bone broth, which I find milder than beef bone broth. Bone broth is great to drink often, even daily, as well as when you have a cold or the flu. Bone broth is also wonderful for healing the gut, and it's loaded with protein.

I save all my bones from meals and cooking. I add them to a bag in my freezer as I collect them. When I have collected enough to fill a crock pot, I will then make my broth. I prefer to only save bones from organic chickens, as the pesticides and hormones fed to livestock tend to collect in the bones of the animals.

In a crock pot, combine the bones, filtered water, dried astragalus root and reishi mushroom for building immunity, nettles for reducing allergies, and about one shot of apple cider vinegar for breaking down the bones. Set to low and cook for 24 hours. You want the broth to be simmering and thus may need to bump your setting to High. Ladle the broth into half gallon mason jars. Add more fresh water and apple cider vinegar to the crockpot. Cook for another 24 hours or so. Repeat a third time. The second and third batches of broth won't be as gelatinous but will still be tasty. Season with salt, cayenne, garlic, onion and fresh ginger. Drink as broth or use in the soup recipes that follow.

TIP: Bone broth lasts about a week in the refrigerator. It you want to freeze your broth, then be sure to only fill your mason jars halfway to avoid breaking. It's best not to freeze anything in plastic as the harmful toxins in plastic leach into the food.

Sure-thing Food Poisoning Remedies

Food poisoning doesn't always have to be severe, with vomiting and/or diarrhea. I occasionally get a mild food poisoning from consuming bad bacteria from food that has sat in the refrigerator too long, or from eating out. I almost never leave raw meat or fish in my refrigerator for more than a day. And I am particularly careful with chicken, even cooked chicken, due to salmonella poisoning. I consume, freeze, or toss cooked chicken within five days in the fridge.

How you know you have a mild food poisoning is that you will start to get very tight stomach cramping, usually right after eating. It comes and goes, and it usually gets worse over time, when not treated.

A sure way to treat mild food poisoning is to take two tablets of goldenseal on an empty stomach, 2-3 times per day. Also start taking a high-quality probiotic (also on an empty stomach and at least one hour before or after the goldenseal). Increasing fermented food intake during this time will also help.

I take two tablets of goldenseal upon waking and wait one hour before eating. At least two hours after breakfast, and one hour before lunch, I take the probiotic tablet. At least two hours after eating and one hour before dinner, I'll take another probiotic or two more goldenseal tablets. And then before bed, two hours after eating, I'll take another two tablets of goldenseal. If you wake up in the middle of the night, take another dose of either.

As an alternative to taking goldenseal, you can take two tablets of activated charcoal. If you are traveling to a country like Mexico, and get stomach cramping from the water, activated charcoal works great to kill off the bad bacteria. Follow the same schedule as above, just replace the goldenseal with activated charcoal.

Detox with Massage and Activated Charcoal

I recently learned that taking three tablets of activated charcoal about 30 minutes prior to getting a massage will help to remove the toxins that are released during the body massage, particularly a lymphatic massage.

Healthy Food Recipes

Keto-Friendly Chicken Vegetable Soup

Use bone broth as a base. (See previous section for recipe.)

Ingredients:

- 4-6 C bone broth
- Seasonings to taste. I like to add salt, cayenne, turmeric, garlic powder or freshly chopped garlic, 1-2 T fresh grated ginger, and sliced, caramelized onion.
- Add sliced chicken, pre-cooked or raw. I like to add raw chicken legs to the broth and simmer until cooked.

To Prepare:

Once the chicken is cooked, add your favorite vegetables, whatever you have available. I like to use roasted brussels sprouts, broccoli, cauliflower, sliced kale, and mushrooms.

For a non-keto version, add cooked rice, or diced chunks of potato.

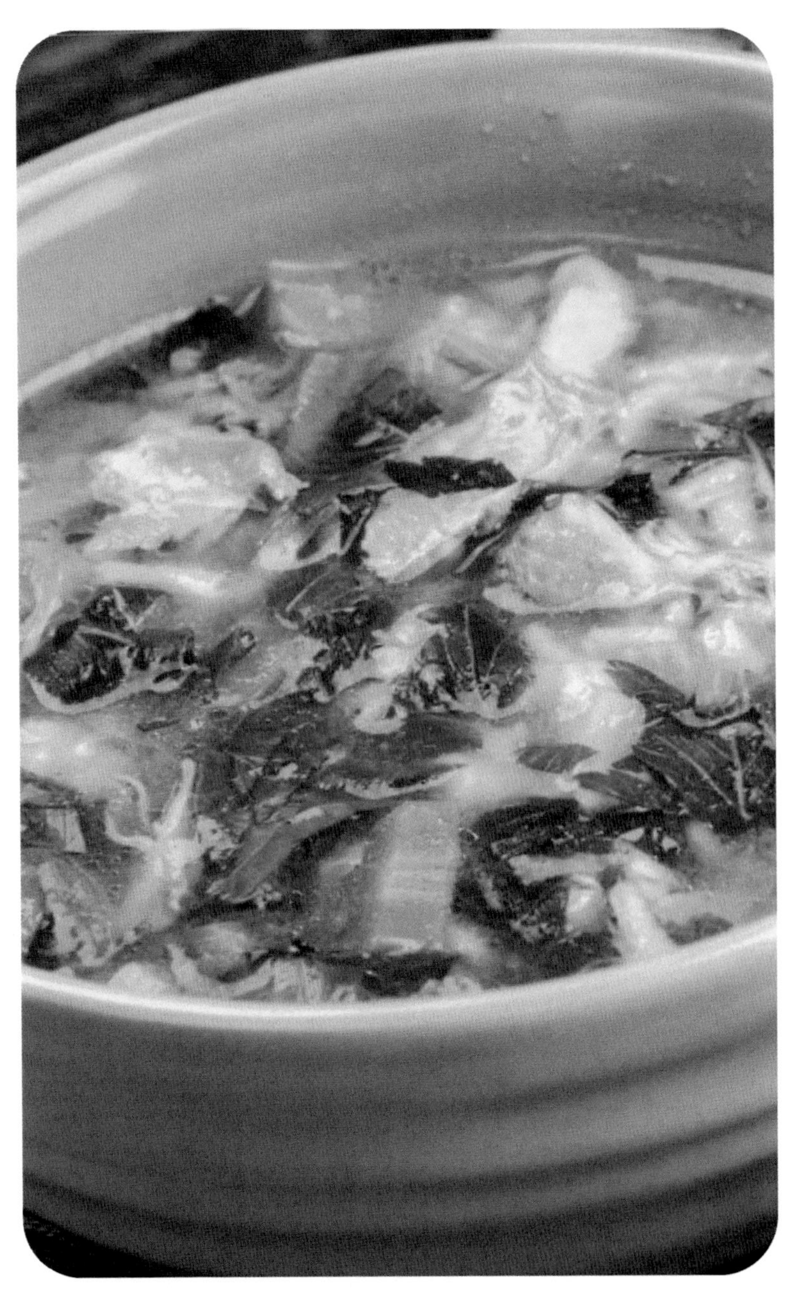

Butter Lettuce Salad with Green Goddess Dressing & Pan-Fried Tilapia

A dear friend of mine introduced me to this way of cooking Tilapia, which is common in Peru. It is so tasty on this salad. Be careful not to raise the temperature too high when cooking the fish or it will burn—just high enough to form a delicious brown crust. Tilapia works great for this method of cooking. I have tried using cod and could not get the same brown crust. Try chicken as an alternative to fish.

Salad Ingredients:

- butter lettuce, or spring lettuce
- sliced almonds or walnut pieces
- fresh blueberries
- 2 tilapia filets
- ¼ C coconut oil

Dressing Ingredients:

- 1 bunch organic cilantro, stems removed
- juice of 2 limes
- 1 tsp sea salt
- ½ tsp black pepper
- 1 T mayonnaise
- ⅓ C olive oil
- ¼ C water

To Prepare:

In a small blender or food processor, blend all dressing ingredients. Set aside.

Melt coconut oil in a medium non-stick fry pan over medium heat. When oil is nice and hot, place fish fillets in oil. Lightly salt the fish.

Cook until a light brown crust appears on bottom side. Scrape with spatula and turn. The fish might fall apart; that is fine. The key is to cook on medium high until a nice crust forms. Scrape the fish that sticks to the pan often.

Fill two plates with butter lettuce. Divide fish in two and place on top of lettuce. Drizzle approximately ⅓ C dressing over fish and lettuce. Sprinkle with blueberries and nuts. Decorate with edible flowers such as pansies, violas, or nasturtiums. Serves two.

VARIATIONS: Lemon dressing: Use juice of 1½ lemons instead of lime juice.

Sauce: I like a milder version of the dressing for this light salad. It also makes a wonderful sauce for meats, vegetables, rice, or potatoes. To make a sauce, I like to add cayenne pepper to taste (about ⅛–¼ tsp) and ½ tsp honey or maple syrup. Eliminate the water for a thicker sauce.

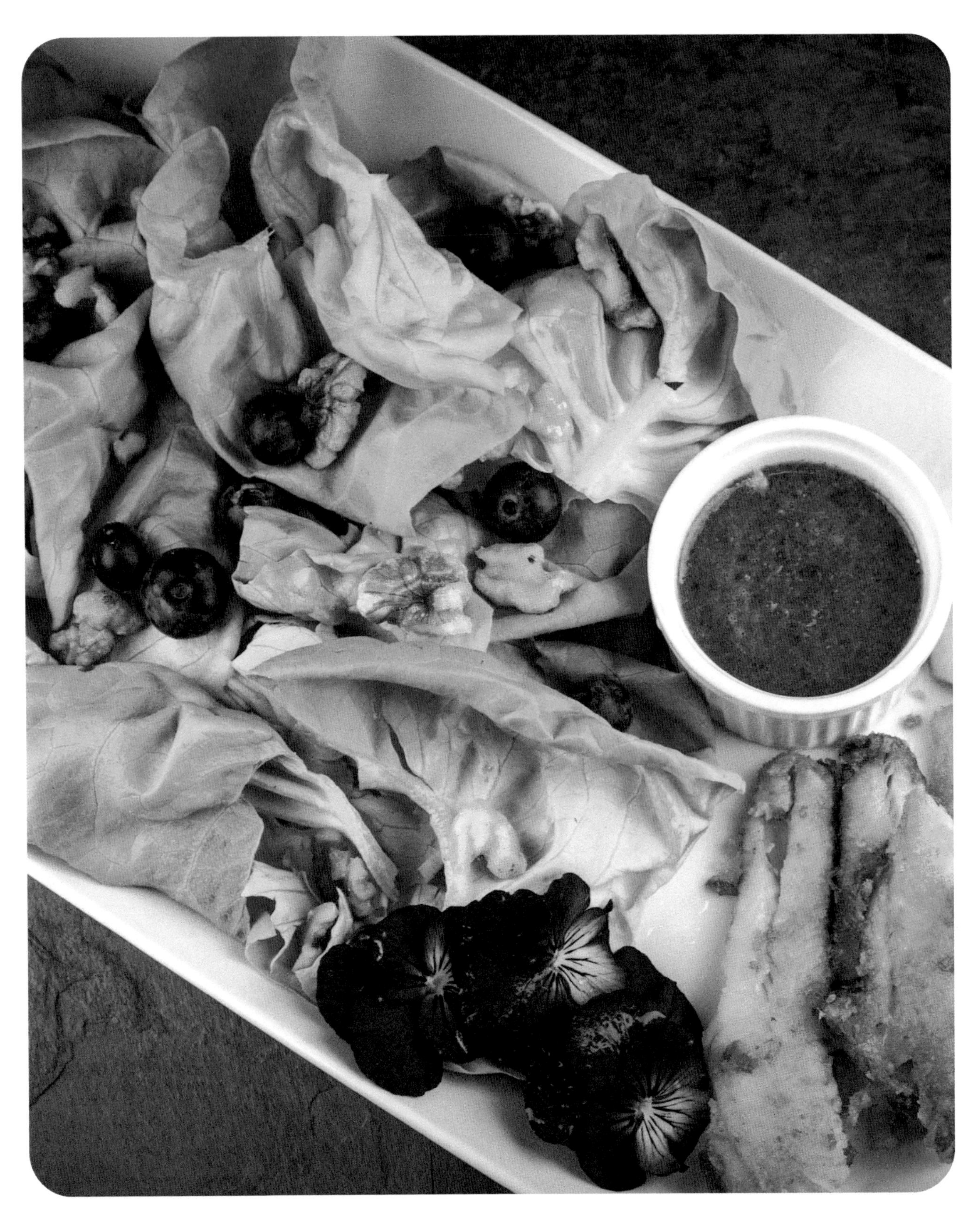

Cajun Seafood Pasta

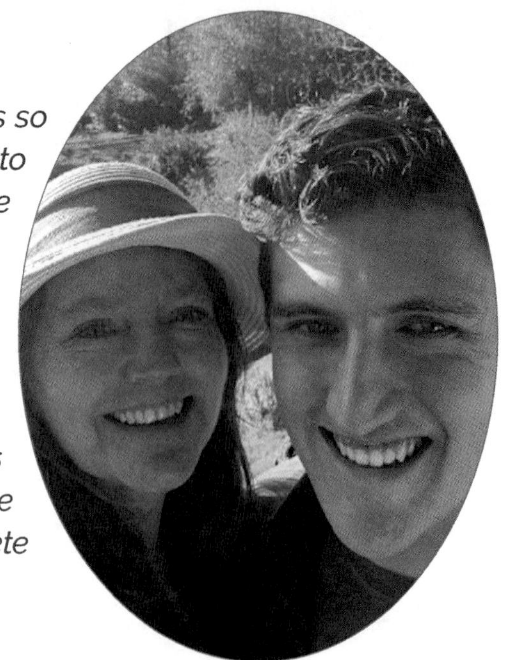

I have a lot of fun in the kitchen with my son Alex! He is so creative and loves to experiment. When I asked him to share one of his favorite recipes, his biggest challenge was coming up with exact measurements for this recipe.

Alex's cooking aspirations began with his high school friend, Ryan, who went on to become a chef. Alex morphed this recipe from his Dad's favorite clams and linguini recipe. He added cream for a thicker sauce and different spices to give it a Cajun flair. The recipe changes every time he makes it, depending on what he has in the refrigerator, but the below represents its most complete form. I love you, Alex!

Ingredients:

- 4-5 cloves garlic, minced
- 3 oz coarsely chopped baby Bella mushrooms (about 5-7 caps)
- 2 oz chopped yellow onion (about ¼-⅓ of a whole onion)
- 1½ T extra virgin olive oil
- 1½ T ground paprika
- 2 tsp thyme
- 2 tsp oregano
- 1 T cayenne pepper
- 1 T salt
- 2 tsp black pepper
- fusilli pasta (or your choice)-12 oz dry
- 1 can (6.5 oz) chopped clams
- ½ C half and half
- 1½ T lemon juice
- 1 T flour
- 2 T tomato paste
- 1 lb. raw shrimp, fresh or frozen and thawed
- (Optional) ½ lb. imitation crab

To Prepare:

Add onion, mushrooms, garlic, and olive oil to a large pan on medium heat. Sauté ~5 minutes, or until cooked. As the ingredients are sautéing, add the salt, pepper, paprika, oregano, cayenne, and thyme.

In a separate pot, bring salt water to a boil. Cook the pasta al dente, according to the directions on the box.

When onions are translucent, add the lemon juice and jar of clams, including the juice. Lower heat to a rapid simmer.

In a separate bowl, mix the half and half, flour, and tomato paste with ¼ C of the pasta water. Mix until the flour is no longer clumpy.

Add to the pan with the rest of the ingredients. Simmer 5-7 minutes, or until sauce begins to thicken.

Add the shrimp and imitation crab. Stir in, making sure the shrimp is covered by the sauce. Cook 2-3 minutes, or until shrimp is cooked.

Serve over pasta. Serves 4.

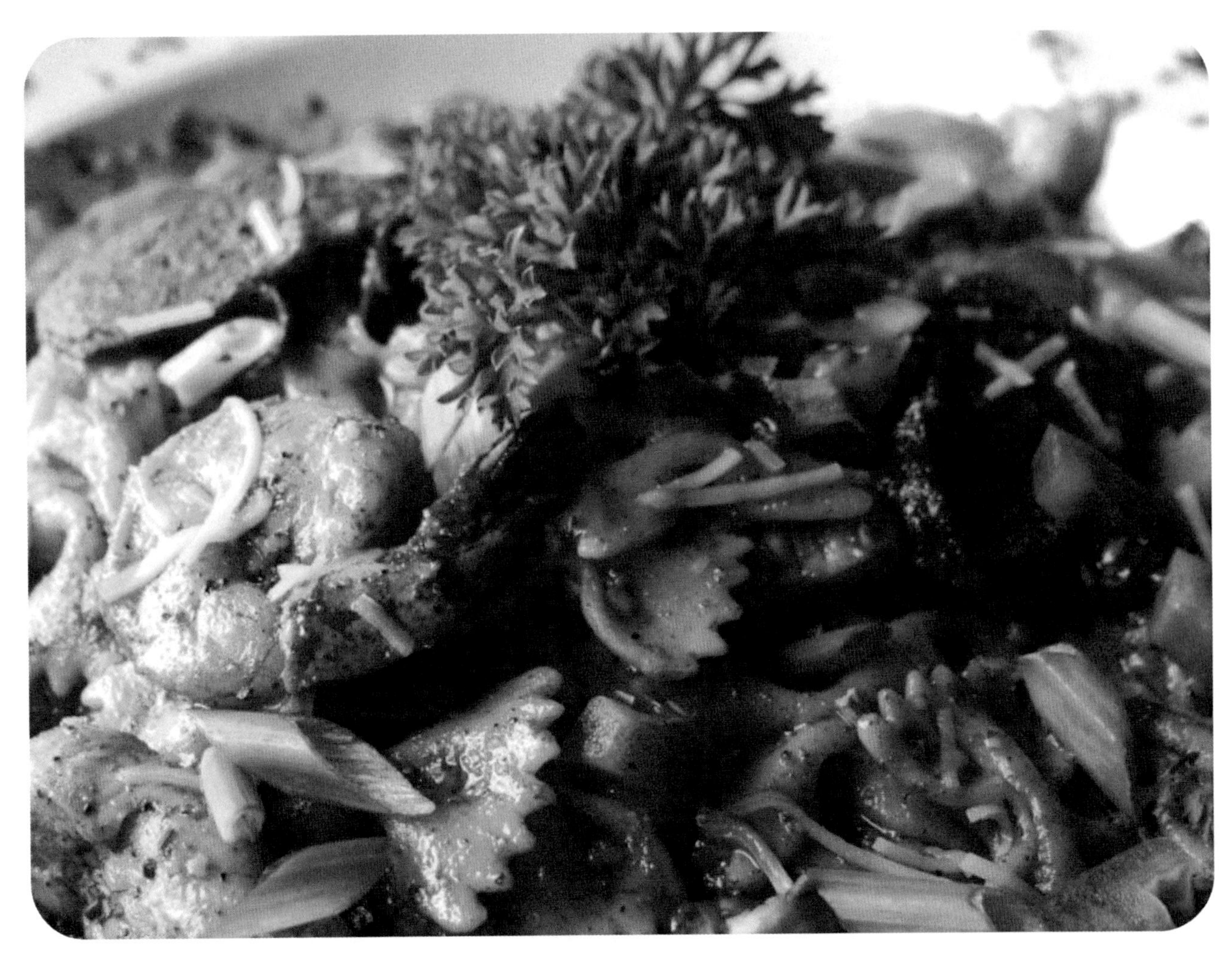

Salmon Seaweed Bowl

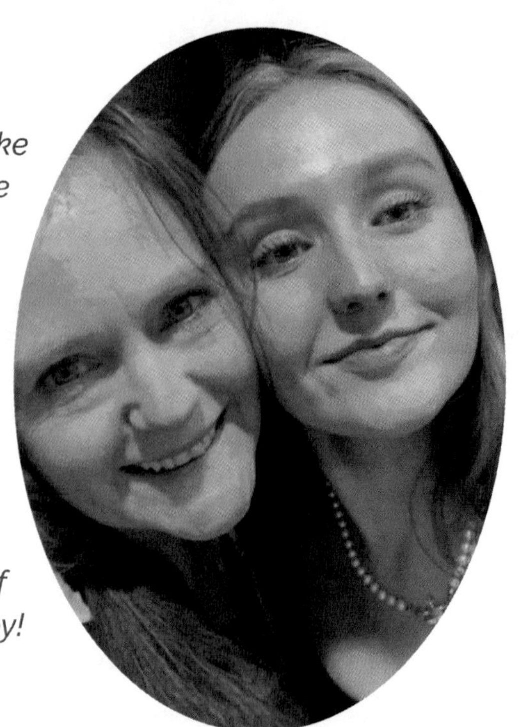

My daughter, Ella, is sweet-natured and caring, just like her brother; she brings much joy to the kitchen. She prefers me, her Dad, and her brother to do all the cooking, ha! But since she's been at college, she has become quite inspired in the kitchen.

As a young child Ella would forever beg me to play "store" and "kitchen." She and her brother created their own restaurant in our kitchen, with handmade menus of their kitchen concoctions "for sale" to Mom, Dad and visitors. Now, Ella lives with four college roommates, and they take turns doing the cooking. This is one of her favorite recipes, so tasty and easy to prepare. Enjoy! I love you, Ella!

Ingredients:

- 4 C cooked rice or preferred grain
- 2 salmon filets
- Approx. 4 tsp Sriracha
- Approx. 2 tsp mayonnaise
- Approx. 2 tsp soy sauce
- 4 seaweed snack packs
- 2 avocados (½ per person)

To Prepare:

Cook rice per package instructions.

Use your preferred method to cook the salmon.

Slice and cube avocado; set aside.

After salmon is cooked, divide filets in half and place one half into four separate bowls. Shred the salmon using a fork.

Divide warm rice equally into each of the four bowls on top of the salmon.

Over each bowl drizzle Sriracha, mayonnaise, and soy sauce, adding more where desired.

My preferred method of eating:

Once fully mixed, place a cube of avocado on the mixture, then a piece of seaweed on top of the avocado.

Using chopsticks, grab both sides of the seaweed, picking up the avocado and the salmon bowl mixture inside the seaweed to create a fun sized sushi bite.

Serves 4.

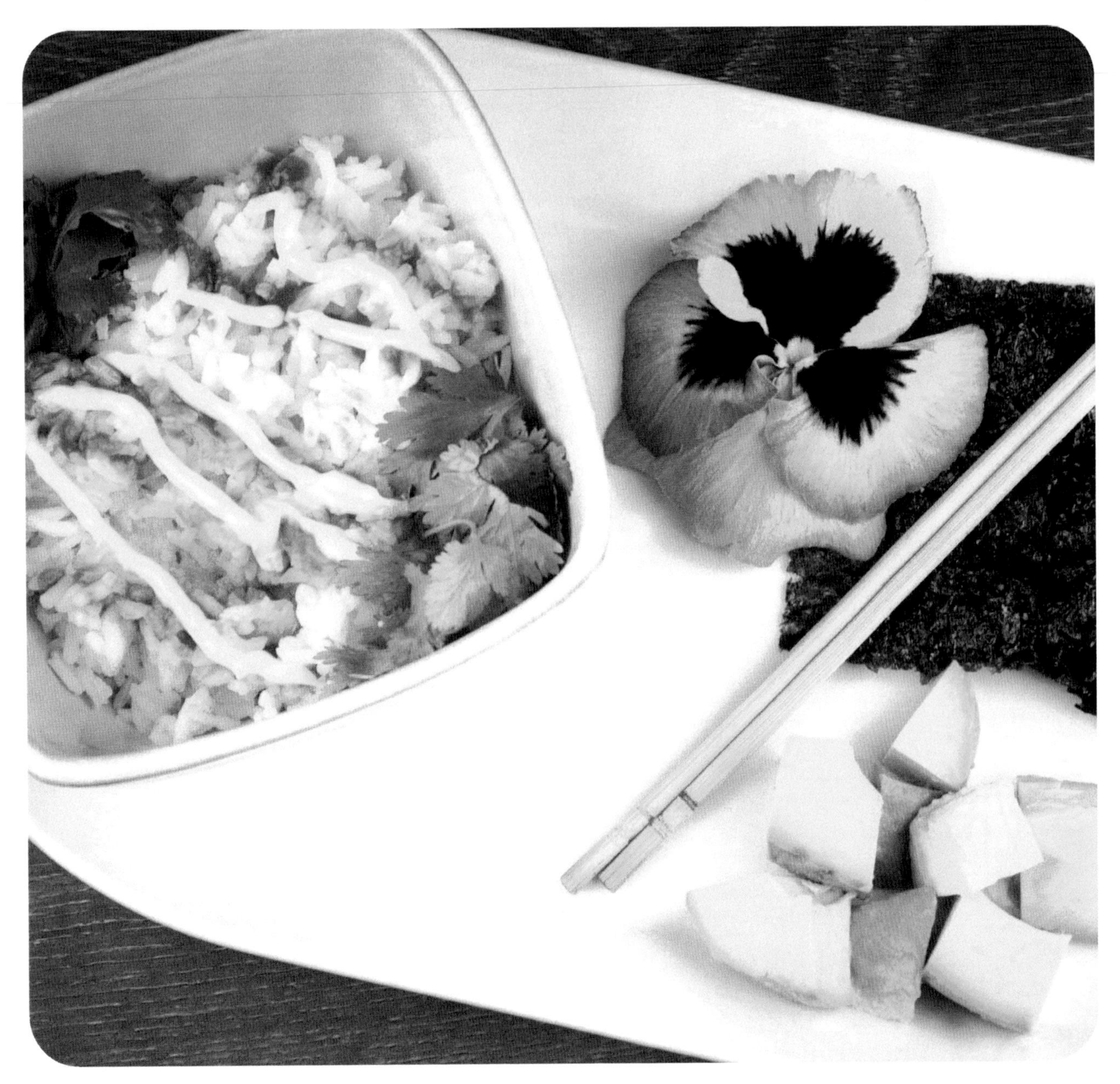

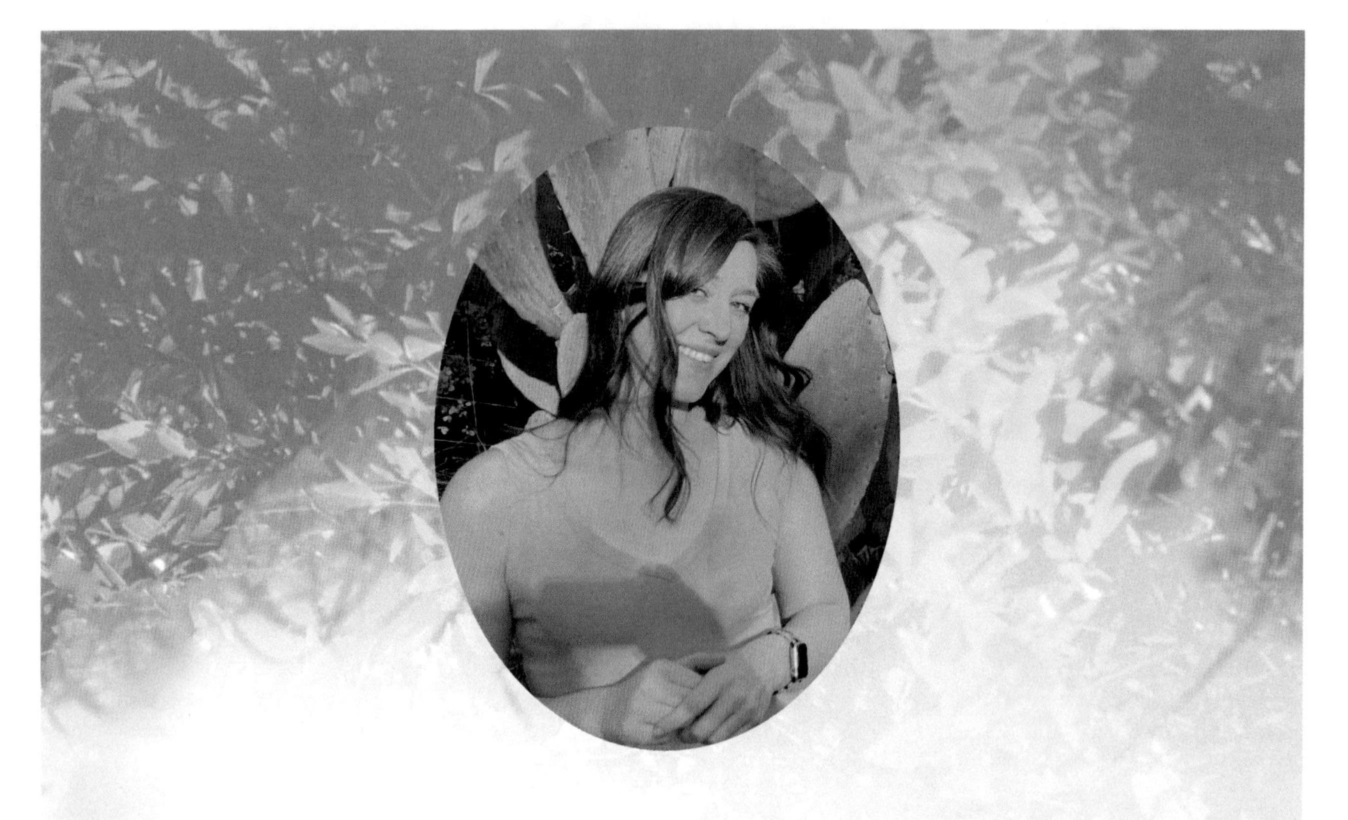

April Faulkner

April Faulkner grew up in Grass Valley California. She was surrounded by nature and plants and became inspired by the Nopal cactus. She discovered the deliciousness and health benefits of this cactus, popular in many Latin dishes.

April is currently a high school history teacher and loves to cook and garden in her free time.

Fiesta Pickled Nopales

Nopales are the pads of the Nopal (or prickly pear) cactus and are commonly used in Mexican cuisine.

Ingredients:

- 3 T grapeseed oil, or any mild oil
- 1 C carrots, julienne style
- 2 cloves garlic, sliced
- ¾ C jalapeño or serrano pepper, sliced into strips (keep seeds)
- 1 tsp Mexican oregano
- 2 C Nopalitos cactus, pre-cooked, sliced into thin strips
- 1 C white vinegar
- 1 C onion, sliced into strips
- 1 C water
- 2 bay leaves
- salt to taste

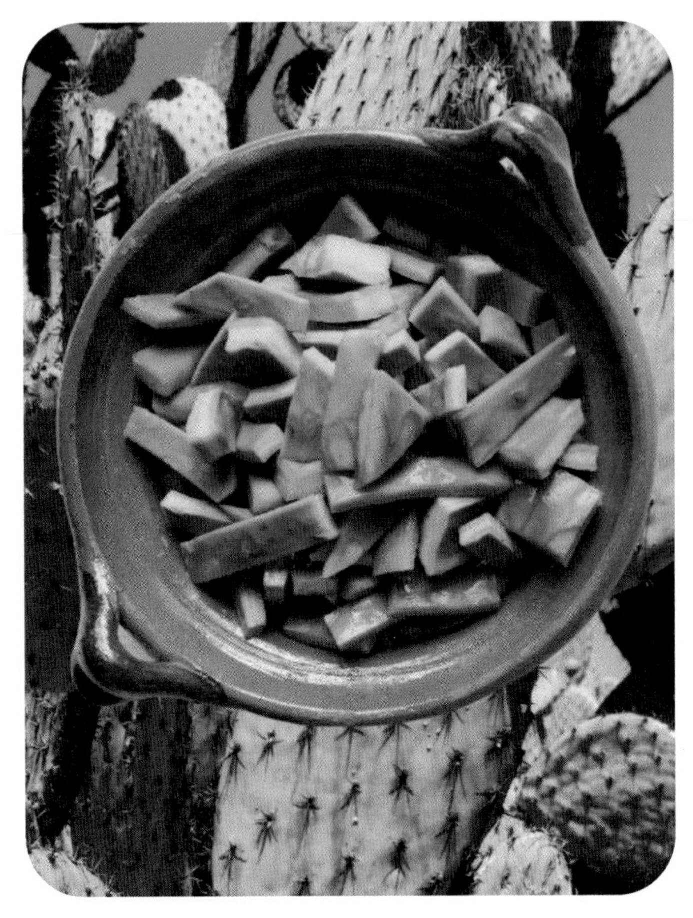

To Prepare:

In a pan or skillet, add the oil and heat to medium. Add the carrots and sauté for 2 minutes. Then add the onion and jalapeño. Sauté for 2 more minutes. Add the oregano, garlic, and bay leaves and sauté for a few seconds. Mix in the previously cooked and rinsed nopalitos. Stir well to combine.

Combine the vinegar, water and salt. Pour over the sautéed vegetables in the pan. Stir gently and reduce heat slightly. Cook just until you see the jalapenos turn from bright green to an opaque green or olive color.

Remove from heat and let cool at room temperature. Store in glass jars with tight lids in the refrigerator for 4-6 weeks.

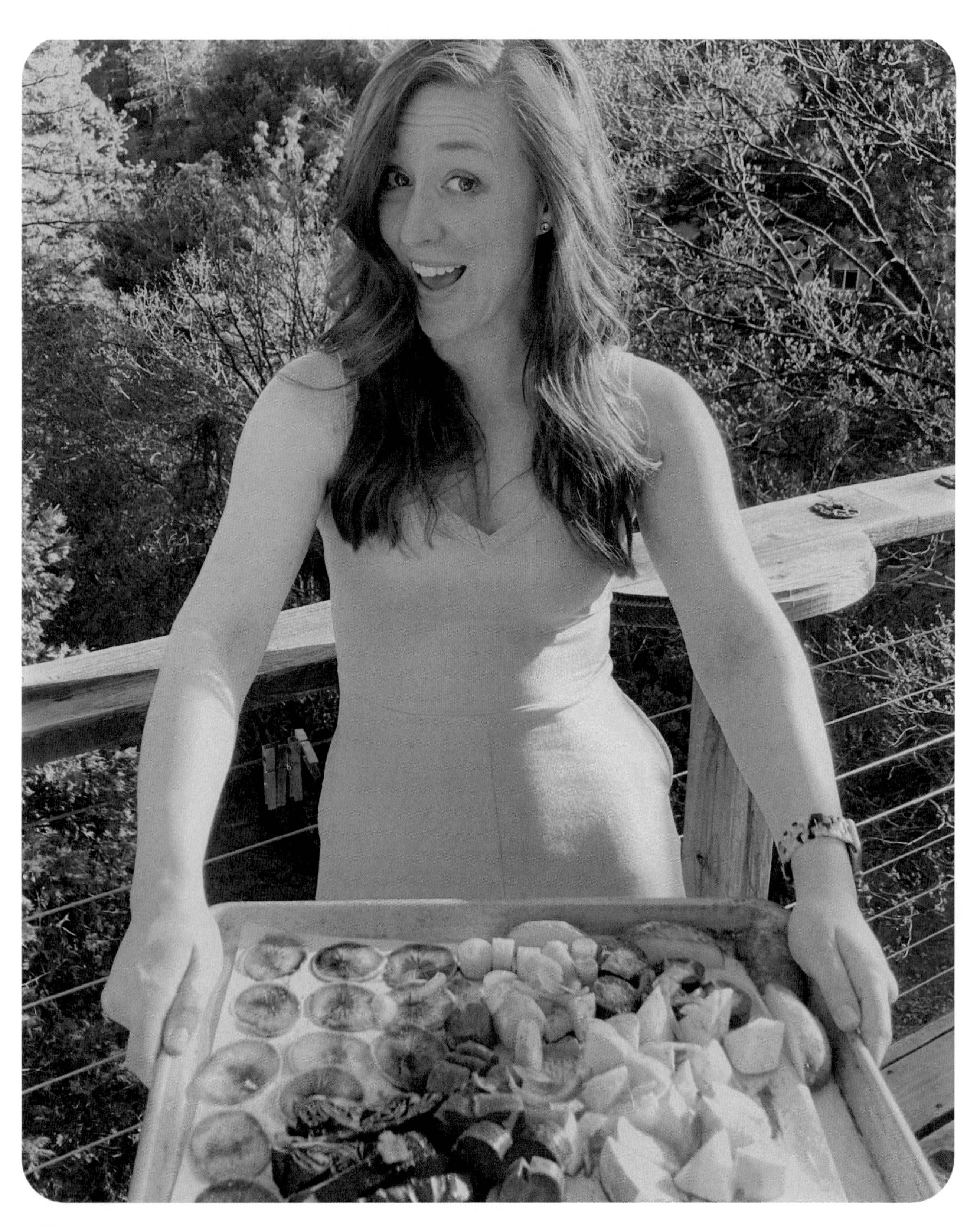

Roasted Rainbow Root Vegetables

Choose and cube your favorite veggies, mix with your favorite vinaigrette and roast!

April's favorites:

- turnips
- red & golden beets
  When mixed together, they create an orange color too!
- rutabaga
- sunchokes
- potatoes
- radish
- carrot
- sweet potato
- non-root veggies I like: cabbage & squash
- onions
- garlic

Vinaigrette Recipe

¼ C each: olive oil and balsamic vinegar

Combine oil and vinegar and season to taste with herbs and spices. Try oregano, basil, rosemary, thyme and/or sage. Add salt, pepper, garlic powder and cayenne if you like spice.

To Prepare:

Toss veggies in this mixture and bake at 450°F until desired doneness.

When you remove from oven, garnish with fresh parsley or cilantro.

Serve warm as a side dish, add to soup, or serve cold in a salad.

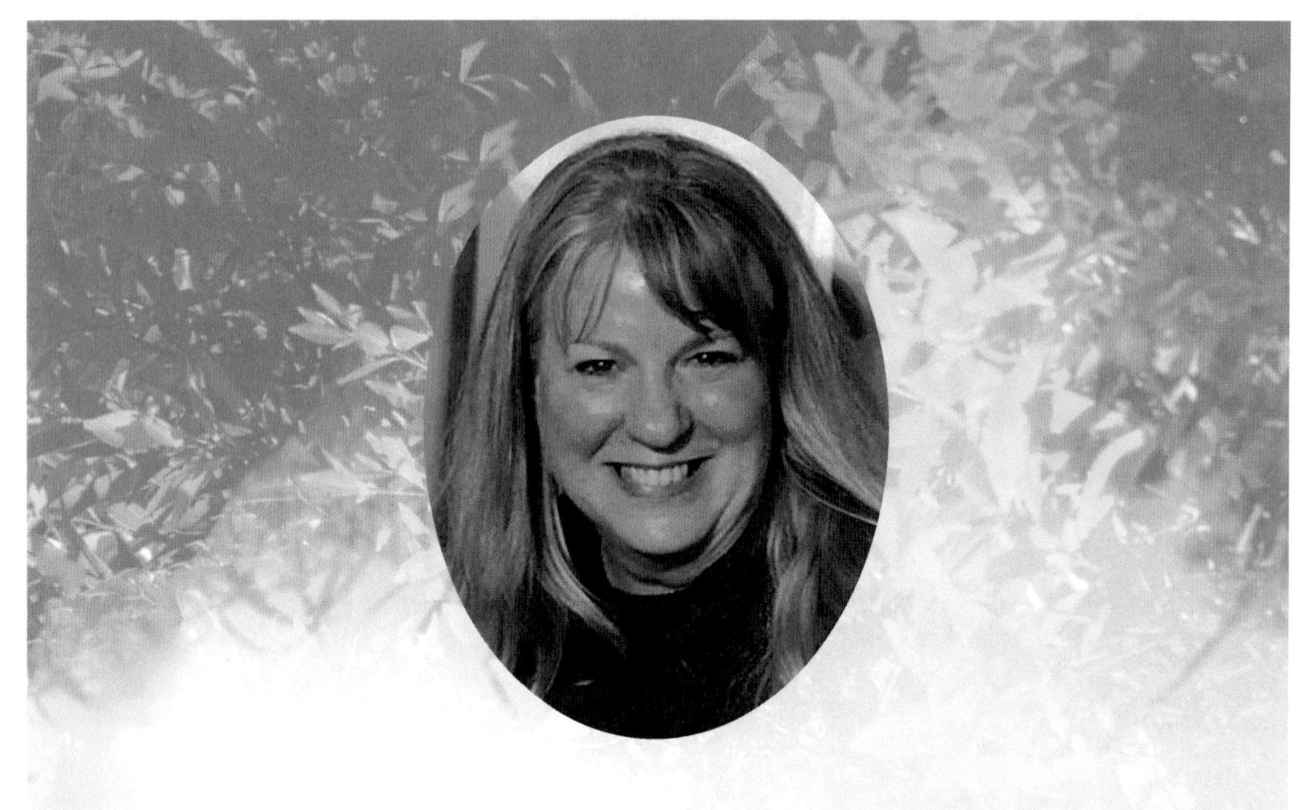

Gale Pylman

I've always loved herbs and flowers, as I grew up gardening with my mom, in a small town in northern California. I went on to earn my B.S. degree in Horticulture at CSU, Chico, where plant identification was my favorite class. While I know and appreciate various aspects of landscape plants, nothing replaces the delight I feel when out in my own garden. This background made it easier for me to achieve becoming a certified aromatherapist. Working with essential oils, from plants grown all over the world, helps me connect with Nature on an entirely different level. I enjoy the benefits of all the body care and home care products I make. Sharing the recipes and teaching others is a new path on my journey and I love seeing the successes of my students!

Nurturing a garden is a magical process, and no time spent in a garden is ever wasted!

Website: AngelsAndAlchemy.net

Email: Galepylman@gmail.com

15

Always Looking for the Silver Lining

Gale Pylman

"It's funny how, when things seem the darkest, moments of beauty present themselves in the most unexpected places."

~ Karen Marie Moning

My mom always said I was so lucky that if I fell in the river, I wouldn't get wet! But my luck ran out in 2003. My dad died, and I think he was my lucky charm. Two weeks later, on my daughter's 13th birthday, I took a tumble and broke my ankle. No big deal for most people, but while I was in the hospital, the IV drip that monitored my morphine broke and flooded my body with the drug, causing an overdose. This happened during a shift change, so no nurses were monitoring me. My girlfriend, Maxine, came to visit me and found me not breathing, with no heartbeat, and my skin was blue. She alerted the nurses, who pumped me full of Narcan and brought me back to life.

I have no recollection of that incident, and if Maxine hadn't told me about it, I would never have known. It wasn't written in my chart and was never mentioned to me or my husband, Jeff.

Several months later, I went to see my regular MD for a checkup. I mentioned I was having problems forming sentences; words seemed just out of reach but felt like they were on the tip of my tongue. Jeff and I had a great time with my pantomiming what I was trying to say, and he kept guessing while we laughed at how outrageous some of his guesses were!

My MD said I had been working too hard and should take some time off, especially as I was getting more and more tired. It was an easy diagnosis; I was working harder. I had a bookkeeping business; there were payroll and other client deadlines to meet every month. Our daughter had been diagnosed with autism. Since my husband worked 50 miles from home, I was the one tasked with setting up Individualized Education Program meetings, and researching everything I could find on autism, in an effort to help her. Plus, my mom needed a lot of support and help now that my dad was gone.

One day I decided that I absolutely couldn't make it out to see my clients. I stayed in bed—and was unable to get up for over a year. I was way past bone-tired. My body wasn't speaking to me and I didn't know what was going on. I was in a lot of pain, all over my body, especially in my back and on the outside of my thighs. Running water from the shower hurt.

I am a voracious reader, but I became unable to hold up a book or concentrate enough to read, or even watch TV. I didn't cry, I was too tired, and my emotions had switched off. I could barely feed myself, yet I started gaining weight.

The diagnosis finally arrived: fibromyalgia. Not very specific, but I was given a lot of prescriptions: for depression, acid reflux, pain, and meds for the side effects of other medications.

I realized that if I was going to have a chance at getting better, Western medicine wasn't going to help me enough. So I would make myself sit at my computer and write notes about the information I found on the internet because I couldn't remember anything. Yes, my memory got fuzzy, and I lost a lot of short-term and long-term resources, seemingly random and definitely worse over time.

My husband took over the household chores and cooked for all of us, including my mom, in addition to working so far from home. We had a wonderful housekeeper, Margie, who kept us sanitary! My mom helped by running errands, picking up our daughter after school, and taking care of her until Jeff arrived home from work.

After more than a year, my energy began to return, albeit very slowly. I had gained 90 pounds. My mind started to function better, so I was at least able to read gardening magazines. A friend gave me the book, *When Sleeping Beauty Wakes Up*, by Patt Lynd-Kyle. I found out that only 10% of people diagnosed with fibromyalgia recover, and I determined that I was going to be included in that number!

We were living in Grass Valley. I was adamant that I would get better and started researching alternative solutions. I needed to make my soul happy again, so I started a flower garden and located it in a sunny area about 500 feet from our house. It was exhausting for me to even get there. Once I did, I crawled on my hands and knees between the rows to weed and till the soil with a hand trowel because, believe it or not, it felt good! I really don't have any idea how much time I spent in that garden, but I would fall asleep between the rows of sunflowers—they were tall and offered the most shade. When I woke up, I would make my way back to the house, shower, and go to bed.

After a couple of seasons of this, I began another garden that was much closer to the house, and shaded by a beautiful old tree, whom I named "Grandmother Oak." This became my fairy garden, and Jeff helped me create it. We still love spending time there! It is such a magical place, filled with a variety of plants and fun statuary.

It was in the fairy garden, that my friend, Luci, also an aromatherapist, introduced me to essential oils, and I began my studies in aromatherapy. I tried various combinations of oils and was so impressed by the results; they helped alleviate many of my fibromyalgia symptoms. I then started weaning myself off most of the medications my doctor had prescribed.

At this point, I realized I was taking 12 different medications every day! I was disgusted—at my doctor, who only increased the number and dosage of pills, and at myself for allowing this to happen. I persevered, finding more ways to incorporate essential oils daily, eating local farm-fresh foods, drinking herbal teas, and napping in my gardens. And I got better! I'm still not 100%, but I'm okay with that because now I have so much more empathy and understanding for others who have also suffered from immune disorders.

The essential oils made such a dramatic difference in my life that I began my business, "Angels and Alchemy," using the power of essential oils combined with basic, natural ingredients to make personal body care products. I'm now sharing my experiences with others through writing and teaching. I hope you enjoy the magic of essential oils as much as I do!

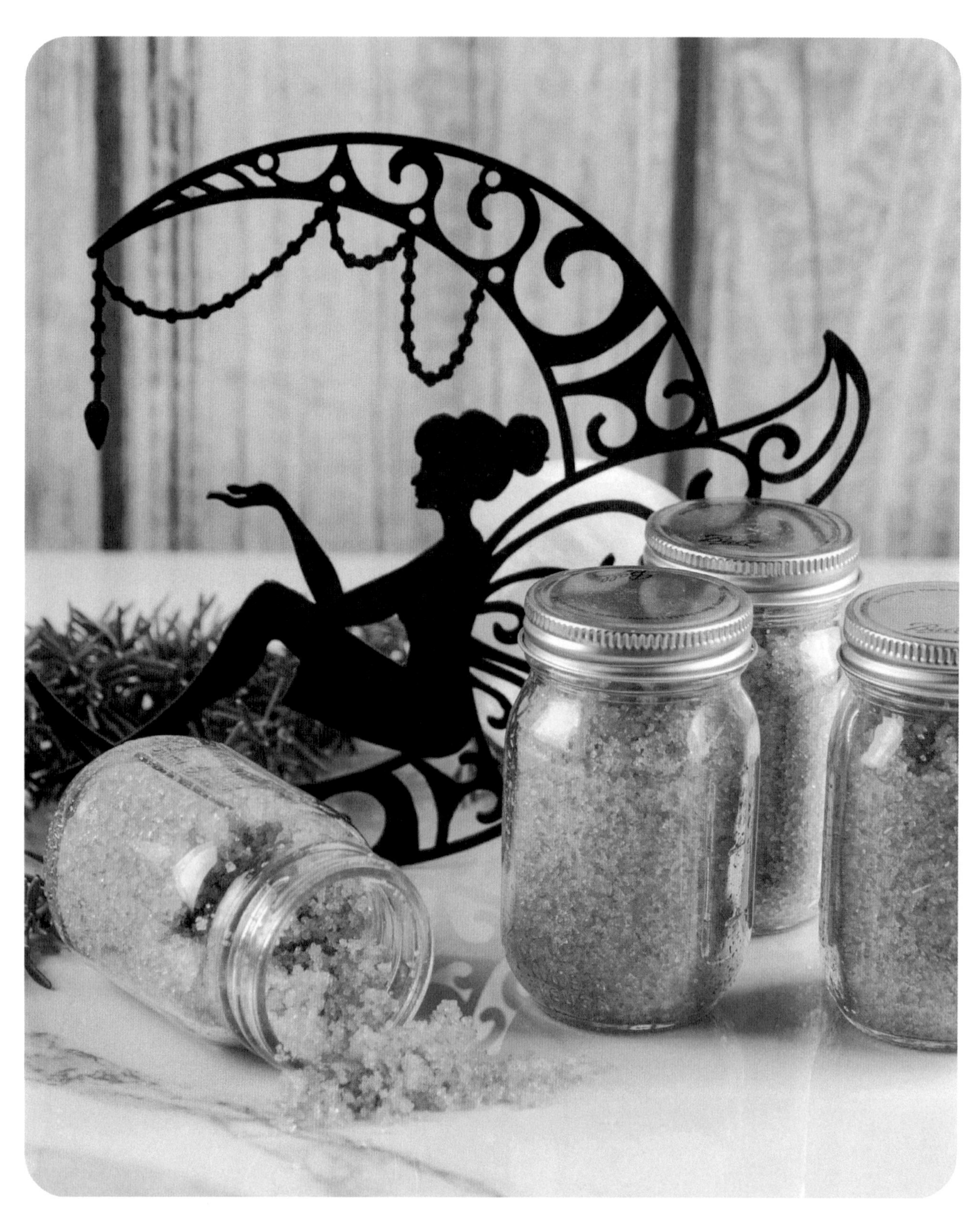

BODY CARE & AROMATHERAPY

No Sweat Sugar Scrub

What's so great about sugar scrubs? The short answer is EVERYTHING!

Sugar scrubs are so useful as a natural body scrub. Gentle enough for most sensitive skin, a sugar scrub will help exfoliate, breaking down layers of dead skin and smoothing the surface. It removes toxins that have built up from UV rays, pollution, sweat, and plain old dirt. The oils in this recipe will rehydrate, moisturize and nourish your skin.

While I don't recommend using a sugar scrub on your face (the sugar granules can put tears in your skin and possibly cause scarring), DO use it for your lips! It will taste and smell wonderful, leaving your lips plump and glowing!

Believe it or not, I get the most benefit from my sugar scrub by using it on my underarms! The sugar won't burn like a salt scrub would if I accidentally cut myself when shaving. The essential oils effectively remove bacteria, and the carrier oils moisturize the skin. With daily use, I have found my armpits don't smell, and I only use my homemade body powder as a deodorant.

FYI: Apocrine glands, located in our underarms, release a fluid (sweat) when our body temp goes up, and when combined with bacteria, residue from deodorant, or other impurities, it causes our armpits to smell.

FYI: Smell your armpits *after* your shower. Often, we rush through our bathing time and don't get really clean. If your underarms (or bath towel) are still stinky, you *need* a sugar scrub!

FYI: I always make a large batch because sugar scrubs make great gifts! I also put a generous quantity aside in a recycled glass jar so I can refill my own scrub easily.

FYI: You can mix different types of sugars. I choose organic ones in different colors because I love the way it looks when blended.

No Sweat Sugar Scrub Recipe

To use: apply a sufficient amount of sugar scrub to wet skin over your entire body, massaging in a circular motion to allow the granules to remove dead skin cells and buff surface of skin. Rinse off well, pat skin dry. Makes approximately 3 cups of sugar scrub.

Gather:

(8) 4 oz. Mason jars or other decorative jars (preferably glass).
Enough to hold up to 3 cups total dry ingredients

1 C granulated cane sugar, organic

1 C coconut palm sugar, organic

1 C turbinado (raw) sugar, organic

30 mls apricot kernel oil

30 mls grapeseed oil

36 drops essential oils*

**I love a mixture of lemon, lavender, and rosemary, or eucalyptus, peppermint and orange, which are major bacteria busters! I urge you to PLAY! Try different combinations and use whatever blend smells wonderful to you.*

To Prepare:

1. Using a large glass or metal bowl, combine all sugars and mix together.
2. Add both apricot kernel and grapeseed oils to the sugars and stir thoroughly. The consistency you want is to squeeze a handful and have it hold its shape. If too moist, add more sugar; if too dry, add a tiny bit more of either Grapeseed or Apricot Kernel oil.
3. Add 36 drops of essential oil(s) to mixture and stir well again. The sugar will absorb all the wet ingredients, without becoming clumpy or dissolving into a paste.
4. Fill containers with blended sugars. *Ta Da!*
5. Add labels, ribbons, etc. as desired.

Salt of the Earth Scrubs

Salt scrubs are very similar to sugar scrubs, and so very easy to make! They have entirely different uses however, and I always seem to breathe easier and become more relaxed when I indulge in using my home-made salt scrubs.

My favorite time to use a salt scrub is after a day on my feet! I fill a foot bath with warm water, add bath salts and small river rocks and sit outside on my porch, soaking my feet, watching the grass (and the weeds, lol) grow. Adding small rocks or marbles to the foot bath is a built-in massaging technique! Plus, they are fun to play with – figuring out which ones can you pick up with your toes is actually a great stretching exercise for your feet.

Using a variety of types of salt is beneficial, whether you are wanting to soothe and smooth your knees, elbows, and/or heels, or washing deep grease and dirt from your hands. Each type of salt has different shaped crystals, and those semi-sharp points are what does the scrubbing work. Be aware of those points when using a salt scrub on your body – do a small spot first and see how your body reacts – keep away from sensitive skin (especially your face, neck and decolletage), and never scrub too hard; be nice to yourself! You will be rewarded with exfoliating hard, dead skins cells, and enjoy glowing skin, that is feeling fresh and moisturized.

Making your own salt scrub offers so many benefits:

1. There are no preservatives that can actually harm your skin!
2. The options never end; try different types of salts, oils and essential oils. I have favorite blends for every season.
3. I love being able to customize the salt scrub for whether my skin is dry or dingy, or if I need a pick-me-up feeling, or time to relax.
4. You can't beat the price by selecting common ingredients that most of us have on hand. In a pinch, I will grab the Himalayan salt out of the pantry, and the avocado or refined coconut oil out of the cupboard and toss in a few drops of essential oils – and it's wonderful!
5. A perfect gift for a hostess, birthday, teacher or a group of girlfriends. Combine with my No Sweat Sugar Scrub to make an extra special spa present!
6. So quick and easy to make – there's no excuse not to have it on hand.

FYI: Different salts contain various minerals. For example Himalayan salt contains 84 minerals, while Epsom salts contain a large quantity of magnesium, which is wonderful for easing muscle and joint soreness. Sea salt contains magnesium, potassium and calcium. The benefits of all these minerals help cleanse the skin, improve circulation and reduce inflammation.

TIP: Not only does this recipe work well as a body scrub, but it is fabulous in a bath as well! If you only want to use it as a bath salt, reduce the carrier oils to one tablespoon per two cups salt. Add the same amount of essential oils as in the body scrub recipe.

TIP: I add dried lavender and other dried herbs to my salt scrub, because it looks prettier, and adds even more aroma. Make sure that whatever herbs you add will flow easily down your drain and not clog it.

TIP: I use this as a potpourri mix in my home. Spiritually, salt offers purification and protection. I put the mix in pretty glass jars and place them around my home, shaking them once per month to release fresh fragrance. If needed, I add a few drops of essential oil for even more aroma.

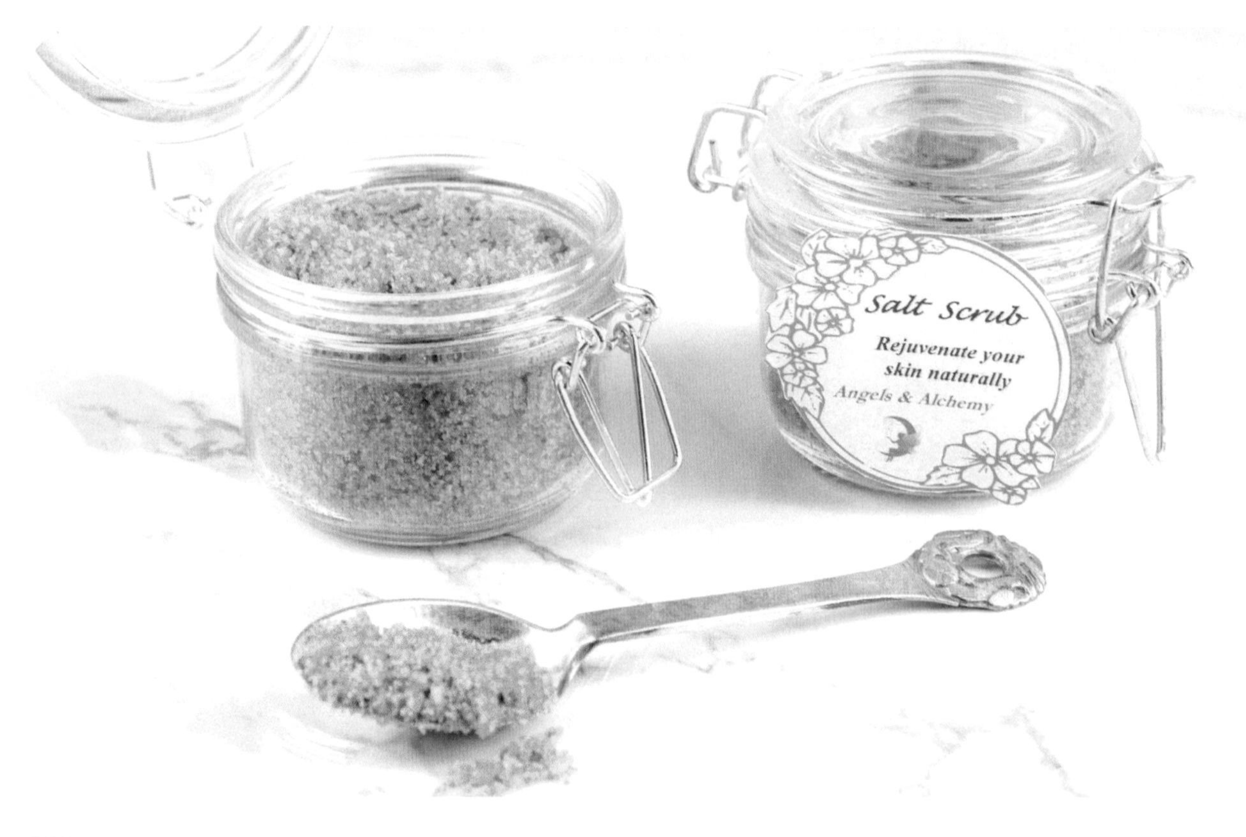

Salt of the Earth Scrub Recipe

To use, apply a sufficient amount of salt scrub to wet skin over your legs, elbows, and heels. Avoid sensitive skin areas. Massage gently in a circular motion, with your hand or a wash-cloth, allowing the salt to remove dead skin cells and buff the surface of skin. Rinse off well, pat skin dry. Makes approximately 3 cups of salt scrub.

Ingredients:

(8) 4 oz. Mason jars or other decorative jars (preferably glass). Enough to hold up to 3 cups total dry ingredients

1 C pink himalayan salt

1 C epson salt

1 C alaea sea salt (Hawaiian table salt)

30 mls apricot kernel oil

30 mls grapeseed oil

24 drops essential oils**

***Think about how you will use the salt scrub: In a foot bath at the end of the day? Try relaxing essential oils such as frankincense, lavender and orange. Or in a bath for easing sore muscles? Cedarwood, peppermint and bergamot blend well together.*

To Prepare:

1. Using a large glass or metal bowl, empty all salts in and mix together.
2. Add both apricot kernel and grapeseed oils to the salts and stir thoroughly. The consistency you want is to be able to squeeze a handful and have it hold its shape. If too moist, add more salt; if too dry, add a tiny bit more of either grapeseed or apricot kernel oil.
3. Add 24 drops of essential oil(s) to mixture and stir well again. The salt will absorb all the wet ingredients, without becoming clumpy or dissolving into a paste.
4. Fill containers with blended salts. Add labels, ribbons, etc. as desired. *Well done!*

Oh, So Silky Body Powder

Is body powder old-fashioned, out-of-date? Not if you make your own! With this recipe, you control the ingredients. I know you will be happy if you add this talc-free powder to your daily skin care routine.

Our skin is the biggest organ of our body, and the more TLC and fewer man-made chemicals we apply, the healthier it will be. According to the Environmental Working Group, women use an average of 12 products a day, containing 168 different chemicals. Men use fewer products but still put 85 chemicals on their bodies. How many products do you use?

After a diagnosis of fibromyalgia, one of my choices was to eliminate as many mass-produced body care products as I could, without sacrificing my lifestyle. I did extensive research and started making my own. This body powder recipe is now my favorite deodorant, and my husband uses it too (with different scents). He didn't like my floral aromas, so I made his with pine, eucalyptus, tea tree, and lemon.)

And one more 'family member' in our home—our dog . . . gets powdered too! We live in the country, and Max loves to find the stinkiest stuff to roll in—I can only say, "Eeeww!" So I made a dry shampoo for him with this recipe, using only cornstarch and baking soda. While it doesn't replace a good bath, at least I can stand to have him near me until then!

Use this body powder generously; it isn't expensive to make, and it isn't toxic to your body. I usually dust my body with it after a shower and definitely powder my underarms. In between shampoos, I will powder my hair, if needed, then brush well. The cornstarch and baking soda reduce oil. In bra cups and behind the knees during summer is a must to help keep you drier! Do you bike, hike or ski? Sprinkle in your shorts to reduce chafing.

TIP: You can make this powder with only baking soda and cornstarch, but it will be much grittier in texture. Our dog, Max, is fine with this, but I like the silkier feel that arrowroot and kaolin clay add.

TIP: This is a great, easy project to do with kids of all ages.

FYI: Kaolin clay is very mild and gentle on the skin. It is easily found on the internet for sale, just make sure you select powder form. It is known for soothing irritated skin and absorbing oil.

FYI: Arrowroot powder contains vitamin B-6 and minerals of zinc, iron, and potassium. It is known to provide relief for skin irritations such as rashes, skin sores, and acne. It is very gentle and well-suited for all skin types, making it ideal for baby care and the tender skin of the elderly.

Oh, So Silky Body Powder Recipe

How to use: Press a powder puff over the top of the powder, then pat the puff all over your body, avoiding eye contact. You can also sprinkle an amount into your hand and apply it to your body. Apply to underarms, torso, decolletage, behind the knees, and bottom . . . good for the tender skin of babies and the elderly, too.

Ingredients:

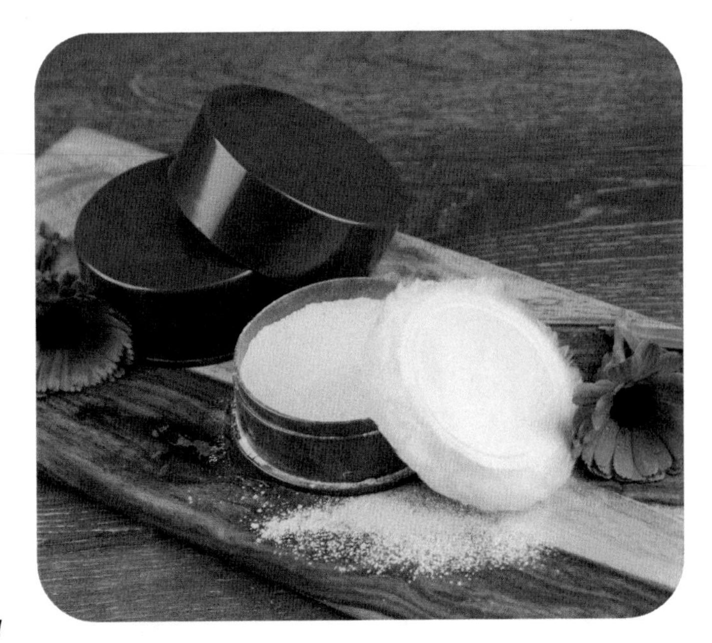

- Body powder containers and puffs or body powder sifters that will hold up to 2.5 cups total dry ingredients
- 1 C cornstarch
- ½ C baking soda
- ½ C arrowroot powder
- ½ C kaolin clay
- 24 drops essential oils**

***For babies**, cut essential oils to 8 drops. Lavender, orange, and/or lemon are a good combination. **For men**, try mixing 8 drops pine, 4 drops clove, 6 drops peppermint, and 6 drops orange. Most **women** are drawn to a blend of 6 drops each of lavender, rosemary, and clary sage, 4 drops ylang ylang, and 2 drops lemon. I also like to blend 10 drops lemon, 4 drops each of bergamot, patchouli and ylang ylang, plus 2 drops rosemary.*

Experiment! Try different combinations and use whatever blend smells wonderful to you.

To Prepare:

1. Using a 1-gallon resealable plastic bag, place cornstarch, baking soda, arrowroot powder, and kaolin clay in the bag. Seal and shake gently to mix.
2. Add desired essential oils to the mixture, reseal and continue to gently shake, ensuring the essential oils are well mixed and no clumps remain.
3. Fill containers with blended powder. You can store extra in a plastic bag and keep it in a dark location.

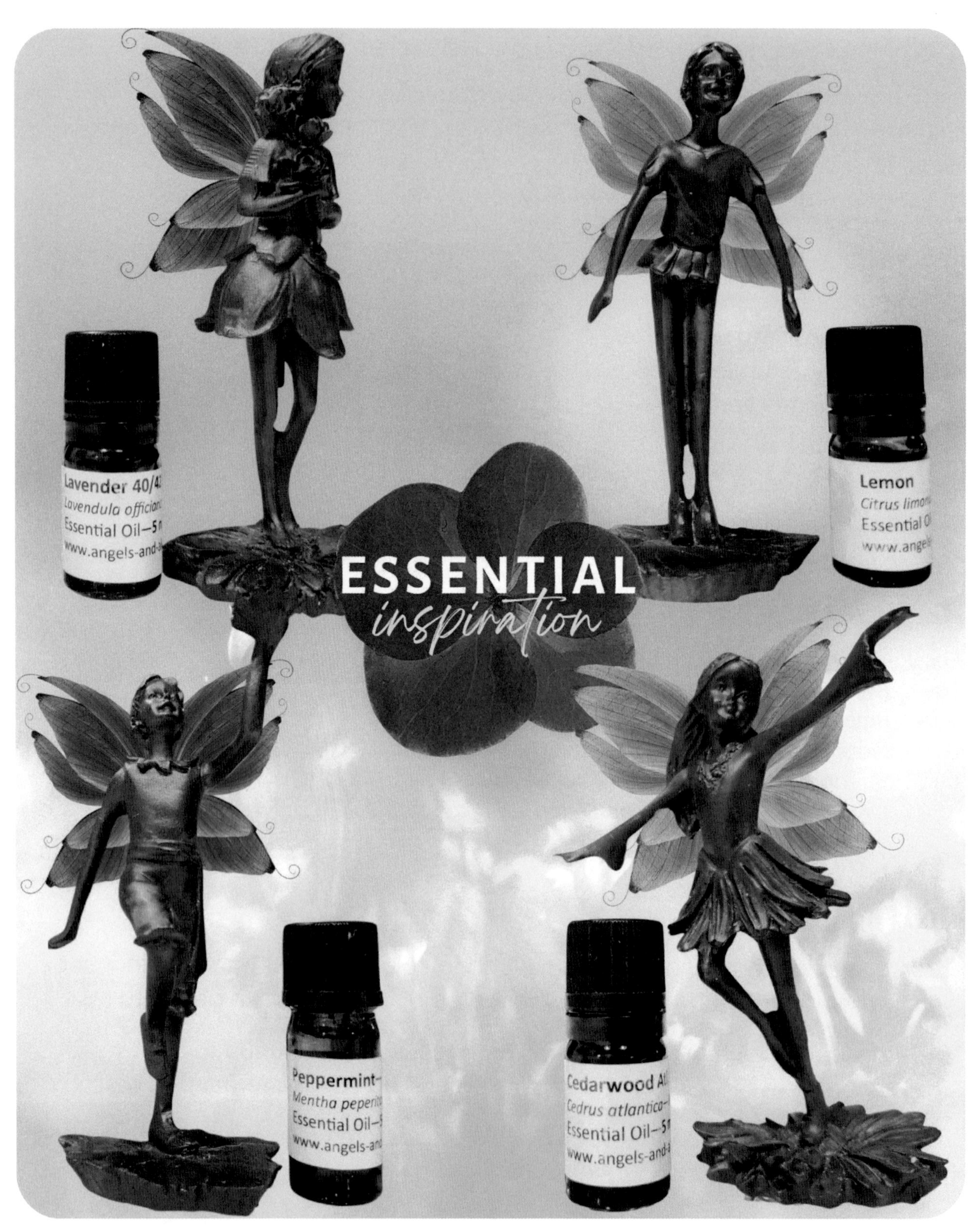
ESSENTIAL
inspiration
Lavender
Lavendula
Essential Oil
Lemon
Peppermint
Mentha
Essential Oil
Cedarwood
Cedrus atlantica
Essential Oil

12 Months of Essential Oil Sprays

These recipes taught me that working with essential oils is as much an art as it is a science! I want you to discover that too, so get ready to get creative! This is all about the "what for", not so much following a tried-and-true blend. If you were in a class with me, I would ask you for ideas on how you would use an essential oil spray. Since you are reading, I will give you a variety of uses. I'm excited to get others input, so if you think of others, let me know!

My favorite spray is always changing, depending on the season. The easy part is that the basic recipe stays the same:

Ingredients:

- 2 oz. distilled water
- 10-12 drops essential oil(s)
- (1) 2 oz. dark colored spray bottle

To Prepare:

1. Pour distilled water into spray bottle
2. Add 10-12 drops essential oil (single type or blend).
3. Replace spray cap, shake and voila! All done!

JANUARY - Blues Buster Air Freshener

I'm still in the mood for warm winter aromas, especially when it's time to take down the holiday decorations. I make a blend of 2 drops each of Clove and Cinnamon, then add 6-8 drops of Orange. If you want to enhance keeping germs at bay, try combining 4 drops of Eucalyptus, 2 drops of Tea Tree and 4 drops of Lemon essential oil. Spray in any room while you are doing chores, it will chase the blues away!

FEBRUARY - Romance Linen Spray

Obviously, a time for love! Ylang ylang can be very powerful, and you might think that more would be better, but not in this case. Although a wonderful aphrodisiac, the aroma can be overwhelming and smell sickly sweet if too much is used. Blend 2 drops of Ylang ylang, with 3 drops of Frankincense. To balance the fragrance, add 5 drops of either Bergamot, Orange, or Lavender. Spray on pillows, sheets and/or blankets. Ooh la la!

March: Foggy Brain Buster

March comes in like a lion and goes out like a lamb (hopefully)! I always get antsy and full of spring fever, regardless of what the weather brings. To freshen up me *and* my office, I incorporate 6 drops Rosemary, adding 3 drops Peppermint and 3 drops Cedarwood. If you want a more spa-like experience, swap the Cedarwood out for Lavender. Sprays are so versatile! I spray this on my shower floor in the morning, then use as an air freshener in my office after lunch!

April: Spring Cleaning Spray

Time for a good spring house cleaning. So many options here! It's hard to choose, but my favorite cleaning essential oils are Lemon and Peppermint. I've found them to be the two most diverse oils; I use them for health care, both physically and emotionally, as well as in my household cleaning spray! Peppermint is very strong, so use a little less. Blend 4 drops of Peppermint to 6 drops of Lemon. You can add a drop or two of Tea Tree, Lavender or Cinnamon for extra germ-fighting.

Spray on kitchen countertops, the fridge and oven, and wipe down with a clean cloth. I use this in the bathroom, too! No harsh chemicals, and gentle enough to use daily. You can also switch out the water for white vinegar, and use it as a streak-free cleaner for your floor or mirror.

May: Facial Toner Spray

May is my chance to get my skin pampering tools lined up before the hot summer sun hits. A good facial toner works wonders as part of your skin care routine. (You do have a skin care routine, right?) 3 drops of Rosemary, 4 drops of Cedarwood and 3 drops of Lavender is an aromatic feast for the nose! If you have oily skin, reduce distilled water by 3 T and replace with 3 T witch hazel. For dry and/or mature skin, reduce water by 1-2 tsp and replace with pure aloe vera gel, or a carrier oil such as jojoba. Sweet almond or grapeseed oil are also wonderful.

Either spray directly on your face and let dry, or moisten a cotton pad and rub it directly onto your skin. This acts as a second cleanser, helping to eliminate oil, dirt, and dry skin cells. It also brings the pH of your skin back into balance. Follow up with a moisturizer.

June: Bug-B-Gone Spray

June is when I go on the offensive because that's when the ants come in and spiders make an appearance. To get rid of them, simply combine 12 drops of Peppermint essential oil with 2 oz of distilled water. Spray directly on the ants, and around the areas where they seem to congregate: kitchen and bath faucets, shower, etc. Spray around the interior and exterior of your home to discourage pests—including mice, without harming your pets. Reapply several times per week for best results. Don't forget to spray and clean the corners of rooms and windows where spiders like to spin their webs.

July: Sunburn Relief Spray

Summer is here, and I often forget to take care of my skin when I am out digging in the garden or boating on the lake. Yes, I know better, but every year I end up with at least one sunburn. I am then looking for my spray to soothe my poor crispy skin. Mix 12 drops of Lavender essential oil with 1 oz each of pure aloe vera gel and water. The sting is instantly gone! Peppermint and Tea Tree oils also provide healing relief, with Peppermint cooling the heat and Tea Tree taking away any itchiness. Repeat as often as needed.

August: Settle Down Sleepy Spray

Hot August nights can keep you from getting a good night's sleep. I have found that a spray mist on my pillow, as well as my face, *plus* the back of my neck, helps send me to Slumberland. Also, it is a wonderful way to help settle down the kids! (Massage onto the bottoms of their feet, trust me, they will love it!) Lavender is well known for its calming properties, but sometimes it takes a village—of essential oils. Try this blend: 3 drops of each Lavender, Roman Chamomile, Marjoram and Bergamot Orange. Sweet dreams!

September: Germ Fighter Spray

Even though my kids are out of the house, I still get hypervigilant about germs as school starts. I use this spray to wipe down the handle of the grocery cart and doorknobs in public bathrooms. I increase the number of essential oils in this recipe, because I like the aroma this blend makes. Start with 3 drops each of Clove and Cinnamon, then add 4 drops of both Lemon and Rosemary, then 2 drops Eucalyptus, for a total of 16 drops.

A must have for traveling! Spray on any surface and wipe down with a clean, dry cloth or paper towel. It also works as a great hand sanitizer.

October: Fall in Love with Fall Spray

My favorite season! I can never get enough of this time of year. It's like a whole month of planning is available for the winter holidays. Lol, it always speeds by! Blend 5 drops Cedarwood with 3 drops Frankincense, 3 drops Orange and 2 drops of *(your choice)*. Yes, I enjoy not knowing what those last two drops will be! Sometimes Cinnamon, or maybe Lavender, or Eucalyptus will dive in. I just never know. Choose what feels right to you!

I have a lot of guests show up this time of year, so I want the inside of my house to be warm and inviting. I spray this fragrance in every room, then leave the container in the guest bath, where it can be used as an air freshener or sprayed directly in the toilet to help reduce odors.

November: Pumpkin Pie Spray

Want your family to fall under the spell of Thanksgiving all month? This spray will do it! Mix 4 drops each of Cardamom and Orange essential oils. Add 2 drops of Cinnamon, and 1 drop of Clove.

I saturate cotton balls with this blend, then tuck them in baskets, and under the pinecones and leaves I use for decorating our home. Adding a spritz or two in the kids' sock drawers will make them happier about getting dressed in the morning!

December: Winter Frost Spray

Need a thoughtful, but incredibly easy and time-saving homemade gift? (Who doesn't?) Feel free to double, triple, or further expand this recipe. Then decant into sweet little bottles you label and tie a pretty ribbon on! Don't forget to make an extra one for yourself! Start with Peppermint, because it will help put a little 'pep' in your step! Mix 5 drops Peppermint, 2 drops Clove, 2 drops Pine and 1 drop of Cinnamon. That's it! Super easy and smells amazing! Enjoy! Now go put your feet up!

> **TIP:** If you are on a budget and can only invest in a few essential oils, determine your main reasons for using them. My two most diverse, hands down, are lemon and peppermint! I also use a lot of Tea Tree for first aid, but it doesn't smell as wonderful to me. (See the April recipe above.)
>
> **TIP:** I save so much money and help save our planet by making my own sprays! Fewer ingredients, no preservatives or additives.
>
> **TIP:** These sprays can be made in whatever quantity you need. Make ahead and combine your favorites for thoughtful gifts throughout the year.

Mindfulness, Meditation, Memories and Magic

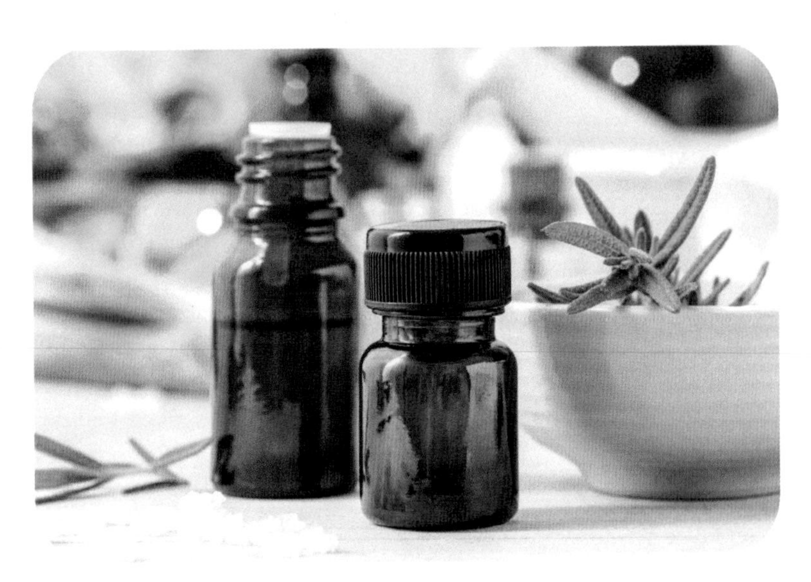

One of my current discoveries for a new way that I am using my essential oils is a fun meditation routine. (It has also been a clever learning trick!) Have you ever picked up a book of inspirational quotes or poems and let it fall open, knowing that the perfect words you need at that moment will appear on the page? I now do the same thing with my essential oils.

I have a small basket that I keep in my nightstand drawer, with the bottles of essential oils all jumbled up. Every time I open the drawer, I am rewarded with the most amazing fusion of aromas, each oil dancing, blending with the others like a most spectacular ballet of scents! Then I allow the magic to begin. I close my eyes, ask the Universe to guide me, and simply hold my dominant hand over the basket and select a bottle. I then thank the Universe for all the blessings I have received, plus those that still await me, and put the basket with the remaining bottles back in the drawer.

Now I let the magic begin. I read the entire label on the bottle, committing the Latin and common name to memory. Take the cap off the bottle and sniff the inside of the cap, not the bottle. (Think of the essential oil as a fine wine; you want to absorb and appreciate the subtle scents, not be overwhelmed by a gust of odor.) Then I focus on what comes to my mind first. Is there a memory, perhaps from childhood or college? Is the scent cleansing or more like a stable base? Lighthearted or serious? What is the image that comes to mind, a person, garden, or maybe a beach scene or mountain path? As I concentrate on how this essential oil makes me feel—even if I don't like the smell—all these clues indicate where my meditation needs to focus. I don't try to empty my mind but find it more refreshing to quietly let my thoughts naturally run their course, and if I get hung up on one idea, I will take another whiff of the oil, and ask my mind to move on.

To help you with discerning some of the emotional benefits gleaned from my research, here is a list of the oils used in the previous recipes with their more common merits.

Emotional Uses for Essential Oils

One of my current discoveries, and a new way that I am using my essential oils is a fun meditation routine. (It has also been a clever learning trick!) Have you ever picked up a book of inspirational quotes or poems and let it fall open, knowing that the perfect words you need at that moment will appear on the page? I now do the same thing with my essential oils.

Bergamot Elevates the spirit, clarifies the mind, assists with confidence and inner strength, helps overcome disempowerment, victim consciousness, despondency, assists in connecting to higher self and inner purpose, relaxing and revitalising.

Cardamom Associated with love, an ingredient of many aphrodisiac potions, may assist bringing clarity to a situation where selfishness destroys love, or the mind is confused and the heart torn between two lovers. Relaxing.

Cedarwood Atlas Purification, assists in alignment with one's purpose, focus, clarity of intent, consecration of magical tools and sacred spaces, centering, letting go of mental and emotional anguish, and gaining a sense of inner composition.

Cinnamon Stimulates mental powers, focus, intention and concentration, opening channels of communication to spiritual and physical planes, open heart chakra, clear energy blockages connected to issues of giving and receiving.

Clove Revitalise and stimulate mental and physical energy, invoke courage, inner strength, protection, healing, stimulate kundalini energy, used in love potions and money magic.

Eucalyptus Purification, healing rites, exorcism, banishing negative energies.

Frankincense Considered food for the gods, purification, consecration, meditation, spiritual understanding, focus of intent, courage, protection, help overcome fear, negative feelings, loss, grief, compassion, and pranayama.

Lavender	Used for inner peace, purification, meditation, protection against emotional/physical violence, health, spiritual love, understanding, mental clarity, spirit-lifting, centering & grounding, love commitments, new beginnings.
Lemon	Increases clarity of mind, refreshes the spirit, energizes, purification, healing rituals, breaks apathy and inertia, compassion, love.
Marjoram	Increases compassion, opens heart chakra, overcomes irrational fear and paranoia, helps gain perspective, grounding, used to promote an easy transition and blissful existence in the spirit realm, protection against thunder and lightning.
Orange	Refreshes the mind and uplifts the spirit, energizes, rejuvenates, letting go of heavy thought forms, opening the heart and mind for love, joy, and happiness.
Peppermint	Purification, mental clarity, dispel negative thought forms and energies, cleansing sacred space and ritual objects, increases psychic sensitivity.
Pine	Purification, cleansing of sacred space and ritual objects, dispels negative energy, crystal cleansing, protection, fertility, birth, inner strength, understanding, healing rituals, prosperity consciousness, manifestation.
Rosemary	Inner strength, self-confidence, mental clarity, focus of intent, to break apathy and inertia, protection, purification, cleansing of sacred space and ritual objects, spiritual awareness and understanding, for memory, to assist transition into the spirit realm, funeral rites, rites of passage.
Tea Tree	Aura cleansing, protection, purification, opens mental channels and clarity, unclogs upper chakras.
Ylang ylang	Attract love, enhance sensuality, dispel fear and apprehension, or negative projections, assists in gaining a sense of self-worth and confidence. Helps to center oneself and to let go of guilt and other negative emotions such as jealousy and anger which prevent one from moving forward.

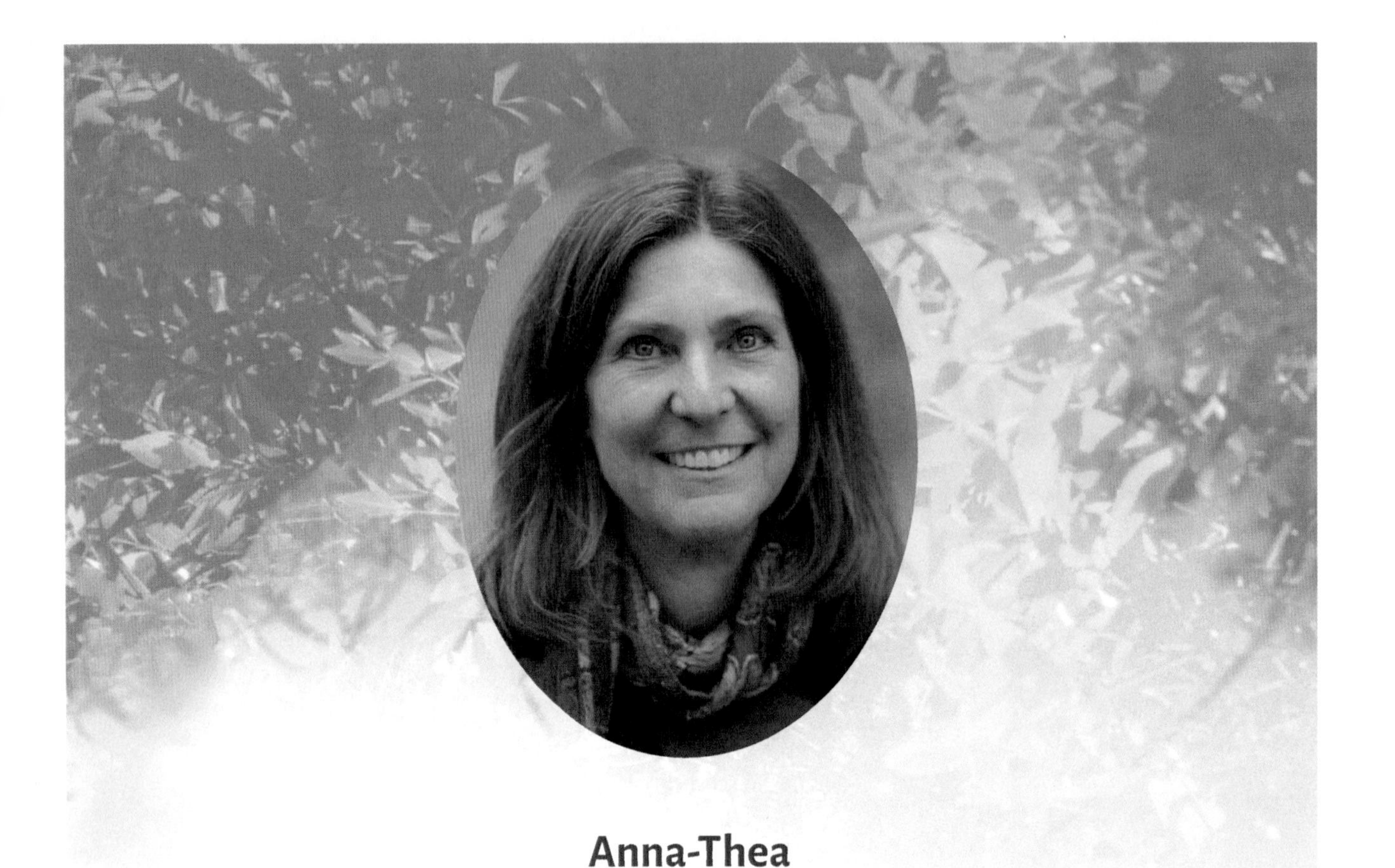

Anna-Thea

Anna-Thea is an author, Divine Feminine Educator, Evolutionary Astrologer, and "The Love Card Lady." She offers education and guidance for people to empower themselves through greater self-awareness. Her online courses and Astrology readings are life changing.

She holds a diploma as an Evolutionary Astrologer and two certifications from the Divine Feminine Institute. Graduating with honors, with a bachelor's degree in Nutrition, she also holds a double certification in yoga as a Vinyasa Flow and Kundalini Yoga instructor, and taught yoga for many years. She now focuses her attention on Evolutionary Astrology readings and Divine Feminine Education.

Using principles from her extensive studies in yoga, nutrition, psychology, astrology, numerology and the Divine Feminine Institute, she educates people on how to reclaim their bodies as sacred. Her book, *Empower Yourself by Loving Your Body*, and her many blogs offer new insights and empowering perspectives on what it means to claim your sovereignty. Her online courses and one-on-one Astrology readings are powerfully informative and experientially transforming.

Website: annathea.org

16

Astrology Healing Salve

Anna-Thea

"Embrace the Wisdom of the Heavens to Awaken and Soothe Your Soul."

~ Anna-Thea

This is a wonderful salve that you can use for many purposes: to soothe achy muscles, alleviate pain, moisten dry chapped areas, and to help you sleep at night, to name a few.

Cannabis has become more and more popular and is known for its healing qualities. This Astrology Healing Salve not only includes the benefits of Cannabis but also the healing properties of other powerfully medicinal herbs. And it includes another powerful ingredient . . .

Astrology has also become increasing popular. More and more people are learning about their Astrology beyond their known Zodiac sign, also referred to as their Sun Sign. You probably know your Sun Sign, but do you know your Rising and Moon Signs? Knowing more about your Astrology helps you to know more about yourself and to operate from greater clarity in your life.

But we are here to talk about a healing salve. So, what does Astrology have to do with it? Well this healing salve is special, not only because of the medicinal herbal ingredients, but also because of the crystals and celestial intentions you'll put into it.

Astrology Healing Oil or Salve Recipe

As you work with this recipe you can modify it to make it your own. Each batch will be uniquely different and hold within it the intentions and energies you bestowed it with. You will make this recipe during a Full Moon.

Ingredients:

These ingredients are a recommended list; you can add to or take away any of them to make your own unique blend. Have some fun with this. What herb is a must-have for you that's not included on the list?

- Virgin olive oil or avocado oil
- A few T of coconut oil
- Handful of reishi mushrooms
- Handful of St. John's Wort
- Handful of dried calendula flowers
- Handful of comfrey root (not the powder)
- Handful of dried or fresh lavender
- Handful of rose petals or buds (fresh or dried)
- Handful of dried cannabis leaf

You will also need:

- A crockpot
- A colander
- 2 pkgs of cheese cloth
- ¾ C beeswax beads

As you can see in the recipe, the measurements are not exact. This is your creation. Make it in whatever proportions you want and follow your intuition.

Place all of the ingredients into a medium to large size crockpot. Put in enough of each herb to fill the crockpot halfway. Then add enough olive or avocado oil to almost completely fill the crockpot. Once you have added the herbs and the oil, then add a generous helping of coconut oil. I recommend using all organic ingredients.

Place the crockpot out on your porch on very low heat. Steep for 2 days outside under the moon's light. Do not allow it to boil or simmer. If it bubbles you'll know it's too hot.

The last two ingredients are: crystals and the full moon's light.

By placing the crockpot outside under the full moon's light, with crystals placed on top of the lid, you'll magnify and infuse into the potion the energies of the crystals and the moon.

I love placing rose quartz crystals on top of the crockpot lid to infuse the oil with the qualities of compassion and love that these crystals hold.

If you want to infuse the oil with a specific zodiac sign energy then pay attention to when the full moon of your choice is. Below are each zodiac sign and the qualities that you can intentionally infuse into your oil/salve.

ZODIAC SIGN ENERGIES

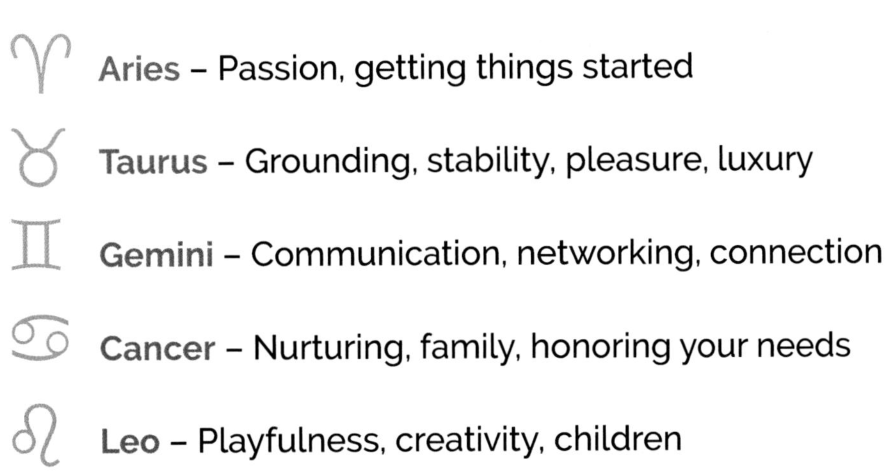

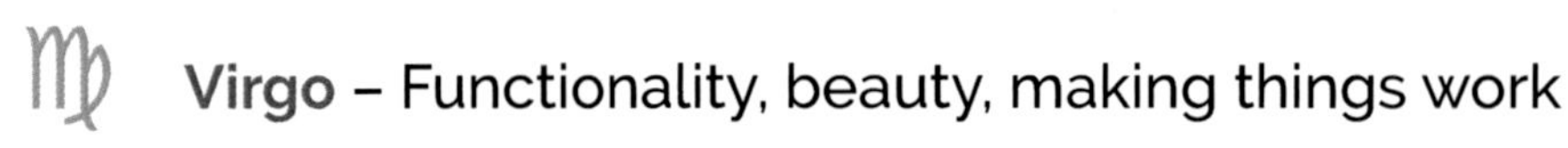

Virgo – Functionality, beauty, making things work

Libra – Partnership, cooperation, harmony

Scorpio – Sexuality, depth, transformation

Sagittarius – Adventure, travel, finding meaning

Capricorn – Authority, leadership, career

Aquarius – Elevating, evolving, reaching new heights

Pisces – Spirituality, expansiveness, forgiveness

Once the oil is made and infused with moon and crystal energy, strain the liquid through a cheese cloth. Then add any essential oils of your choice. This process can be messy, so be prepared.

Pour into mason jars to cool.

Add beeswax to make a salve:

You can leave your mixture as an oil or add in beeswax to create a salve. Adding the beeswax can be tricky. You'll have to figure out what the ratio of beeswax to oil is, depending upon how thick or thin you want the final product. By heating up the oil and adding some beeswax pearls, letting them melt, and then letting the liquid solidify you'll come to the desired consistency.

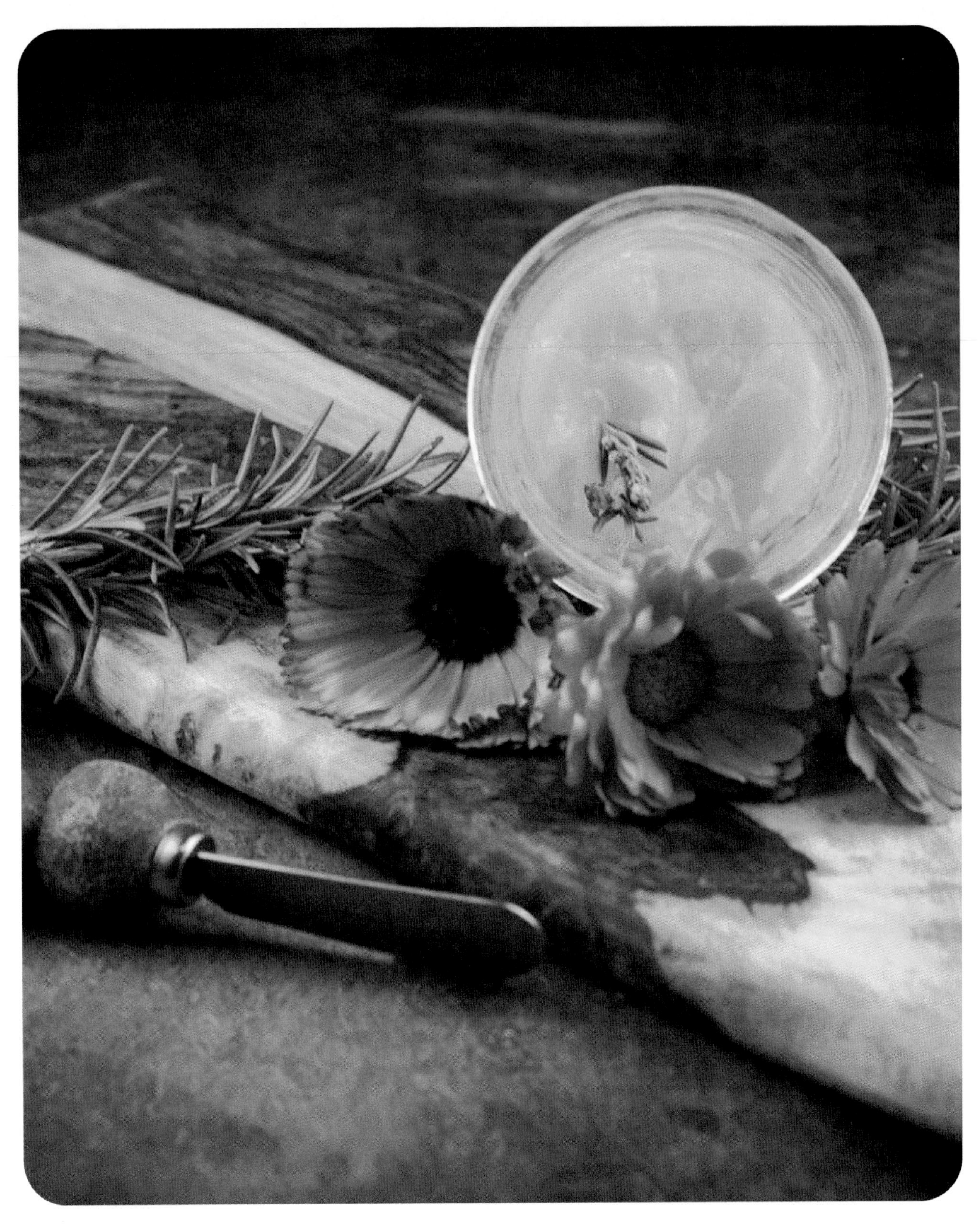

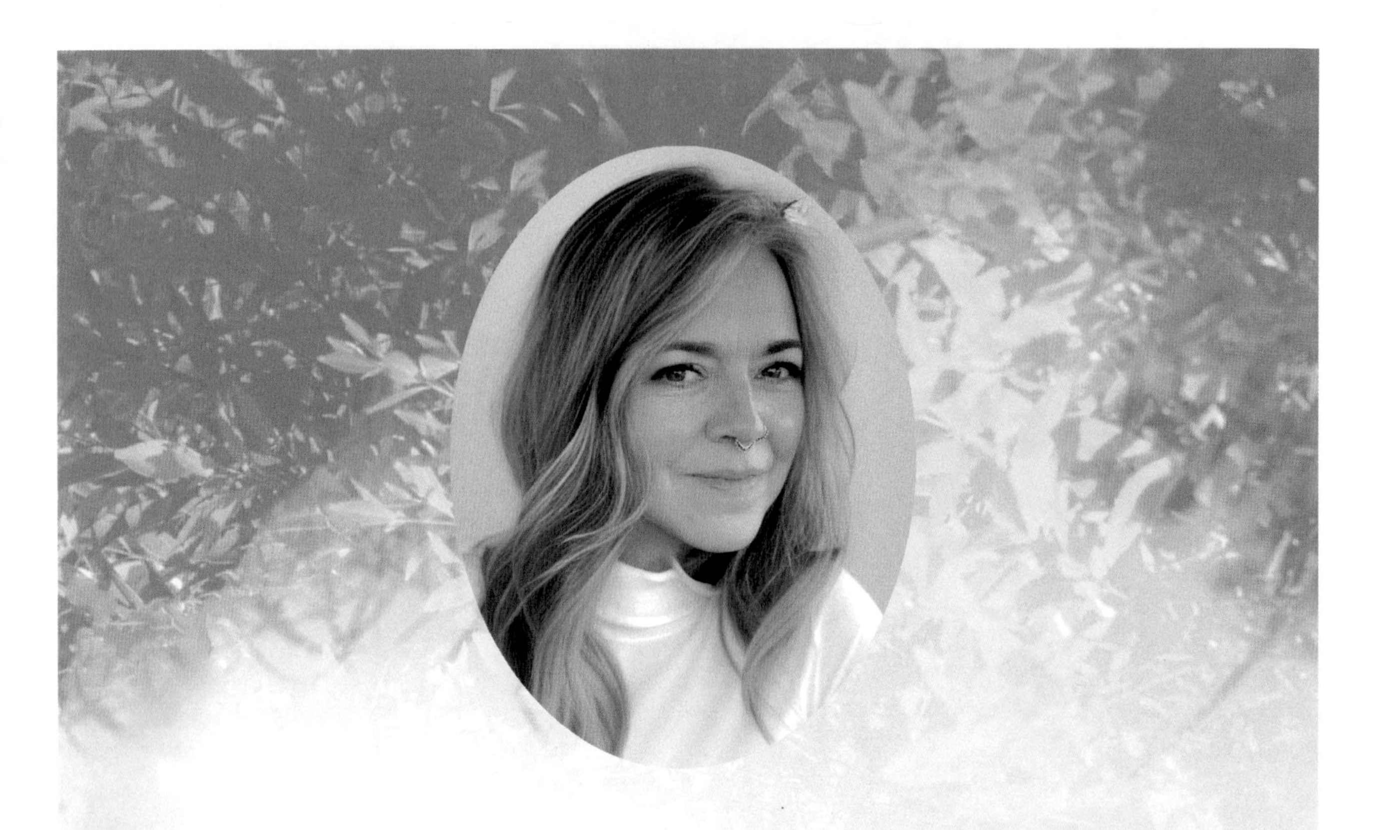

Elizabeth 'mac' MacLeod, PhD(c), LMFTA EXA, AHG(c)

Mac promotes a trauma-informed multicultural narrative approach, applied with self-reflective multi-dimensional expressive arts modalities, to grow clients' understanding of who they are; what their values are; and why they think, feel, and act the way they do.

Enhancing and restoring vital energy that calls on the wisdom of our ancestors and modern understandings of basic trauma-neurology, trauma-psychology, nutritional health, medicinal herbology, and somatic (body) awareness, along with peaceful practices restores appropriate vision and provides the eco-systemic equilibrium that confirms the journey IS the destination. Mac also uses Attachment Theory to decode patterns of intergenerational trauma and identified gift transmissions.

Mac's goal is to work safely and gratefully with clients while building a collaborative alliance with their shadow-self, eliminating the resistance that hinders progression. Understanding how to stay out of emotional/mental spiral trauma-response and instead practice a regulated state is the essence of what it is to claim divine sovereignty!

Website: e2-lifecoaching.com
Linktree: linktr.ee/_e2

17

ecosystem vitality depends on 'partsnership'

Elizabeth 'mac' MacLeod

"Things are not always what they seem.
The deer isn't crossing the road. The road is crossing the forest."

~ Anonymous

I have been teaching the expressive art process to children, through the public school system, as a volunteer art docent since 2004. I have also been teaching pottery out of my home studio for years. And I LOVE that I have been teaching kids (and adults) the beauty and pragmatism of clay for over a decade. Notable in this work is the mirror-like effect this medium has for the artist while working through the process—reflecting back oneself in a kind and gentle way—so that self-awareness, discovery, and integration are palatable and desirable.

For the past two decades, I have been contracted with several local community support services to facilitate enrichment to identified high-risk children of middle school through high school ages and their families. These kids come to my studio in various emotional stages of their life and can present as aloof, anxious, angry, and mistrustful, and yet, somehow, they are all so filled with hope.

In the first class of the session, they usually show up and test me in many and varied ways. A couple of weekly classes in, they are running up to me with wide grins and warm hugs, eagerly and proudly sharing with me what they did/learned/discovered over the weekend. And then we laugh together. They tell me their vision for the day, and we turn on some great music, relax, and create together. I teach them the technical knowledge they request and then hold sacred space for them to explore themselves in novel ways, as they process emotional journeys on the road to self-realization.

Recently I have been meeting with a broader clientele online/remotely. Counter-intuitively, I find it can be as effective as an in-person session. In addition to discussion, the modalities of expressive arts, EMDR, and Brainspotting translate just fine over the internet. Plus, the convenience of online therapy just cannot be beat. Honestly, I feel so blessed to do this work. It is what I am here for on this earth. It is my joyous service, and I am honored and grateful every day.

This is an interesting time to be on the planet. The current three-dimensional interconnectedness plays an integral part in our more-than-three-dimensional evolution. It tells me that ultimately, we are all each other's resource. It matters. I have an ACE (Adverse Childhood Experiences) score of 9 out of 10 and have walked through transformational fire to get to where I am now.

My transformation/evolution literally began with my life crashing down around me. I then made the pivotal decision to reach out (for the first time in my adult life) for help and reconnected with the necessity of receiving it. I have been helped by so many on my path back to myself. And in retrospect, I see that those who have shown up were exactly the help I needed at that precise time. I have explored many remedies to deal with the brain fog, emotional exhaustion, physical fatigue, and situational triggers that tempt me to negatively disassociate and remain powerless after the events that gave me PTSD.

I have explored cognitive therapies in various individual and group forms, employed self-awareness techniques to increase my emotional intelligence, and in general, continue my quest for understanding and relating to my experiences as a sovereign, whole being of creation—not just of reaction. Along the way, I have discovered the wonderful healing modalities of Brainspotting, EMDR, and NLP. I have rebuilt my digestive system from the ground up with whole-foods nutrition, and medicinal herbs. I have begun to understand the mind-body energy connection in a much more integrated way than ever before.

Woven throughout this personal and academic research is the idea that we are all in this together—in a web of existence. We all need each other to self-actualize . . . and this can look like supporting each other. This idea includes the earth, and all of her more-than-human systems, for we humans are but one small part of the whole. We are each on our own journeys of discovery, to self-agency and self-efficacy so that we can then participate in the collective in a self-actualized way for an excitingly new harmonious result.

Elderberry Syrup - Immune Support

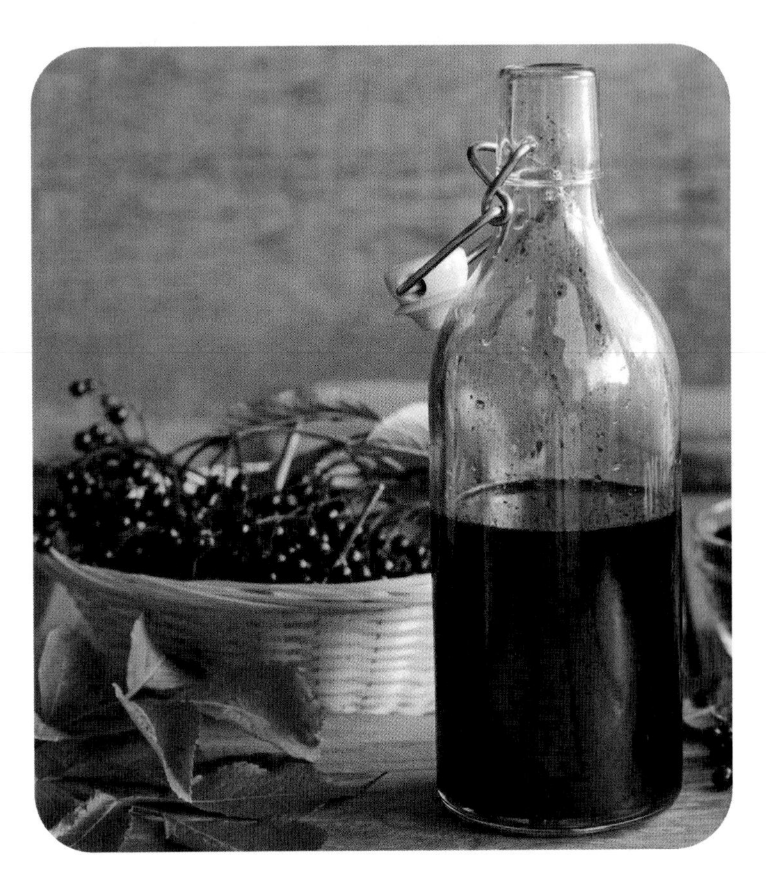

Combine 1/2 C dried elderberries to 1/2 gallon water, in a saucepan.

To taste add: cinnamon chips, rose–hips (crushed), vanilla bean (whole split), fresh ginger root, nettle leaf, rose petals.

Simmer, covered, on low overnight. ***Elderberries NEED to be cooked, do not skip this step.***

While still warm, strain the liquid back into saucepan and add at least 1/4 volume raw honey over low heat. Stir until texture thickens a little. It will thicken even more after cooling.

Optional step:

To make an oxymel: Add raw apple cider vinegar to taste after straining into pan. Add honey, stir and cook over low heat until texture thickens as above. Remove from heat.

I sometimes add a few drops of flower essences at this point, depending on the need. If I am needing energy I might add a little bee pollen.

Cool and store in fridge. (Keeps a few months, but it's so delicious it won't last that long.) I've been known to freeze this into popsicles to have on hand.

NOTE: Elderberry syrup does not suppress your symptoms but will systemically address the cause of them by fortifying cellular walls. The claim remains that taking a daily tablespoon dose during illness symptomology will reduce your duration by half.

Fire Cider - Digestive Support

All ingredients are to taste and preference. You can really play with the "heat" of this recipe, so have fun with it and write down percentages and results for each batch you create.

Fill 1/2 gallon jar to top with:

- 1 large white onion, chopped
- ½ C fresh horseradish root, grated
- ½ C fresh burdock root, chopped
- 10 fresh garlic cloves, minced
- ½ C fresh ginger root, grated
- 2 fresh hot peppers with seeds (your choice), chopped
- 1 fresh lemon (juice and zest)

Add to taste:

- fresh thyme
- fresh rosemary
- fresh lemon balm
- peppercorns (crushed or whole)
- cayenne powder
- cinnamon
- fresh turmeric root, grated

Add raw apple cider vinegar to fill to top of jar (about a quart).

Set on counter, out of the sun, for one month. Agitate once daily by turning the jar upside down. After 1 month, strain and refrigerate. Keeps 4-6 months.

Optional: add raw local honey if desired. (Should make around a quart.)

To use: Take one shot per day or use as the base for your favorite salad dressing.

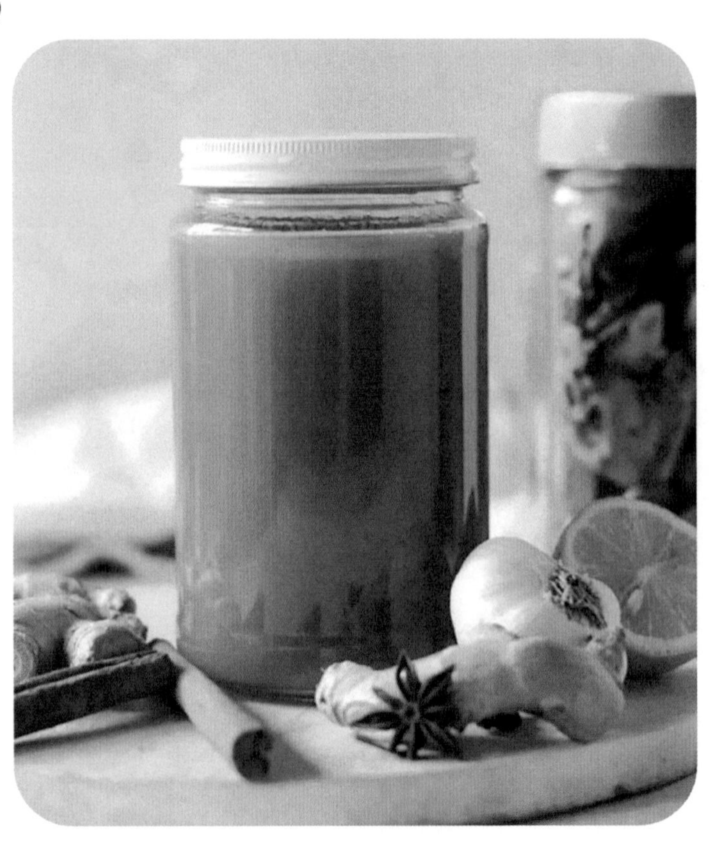

NOTE: Fire cider is best known for heating up digestion. Folx have acid-reflux all wrong. It is not too much acid in the tummy that is the problem – it is not enough. Adding acid before a meal will aid digestion. This eliminates the stagnation of food in the stomach which causes acid reflux. Undigested food sits in the stomach for longer periods of time, and depending on your vertical or horizontal presentation, can irritate the base of your esophagus and cause a burning sensation.

Garlic Tea - Symptom Support & Relief

Garlic tea for vital health and colds/flu/infection. Ideally prepare in the morning.

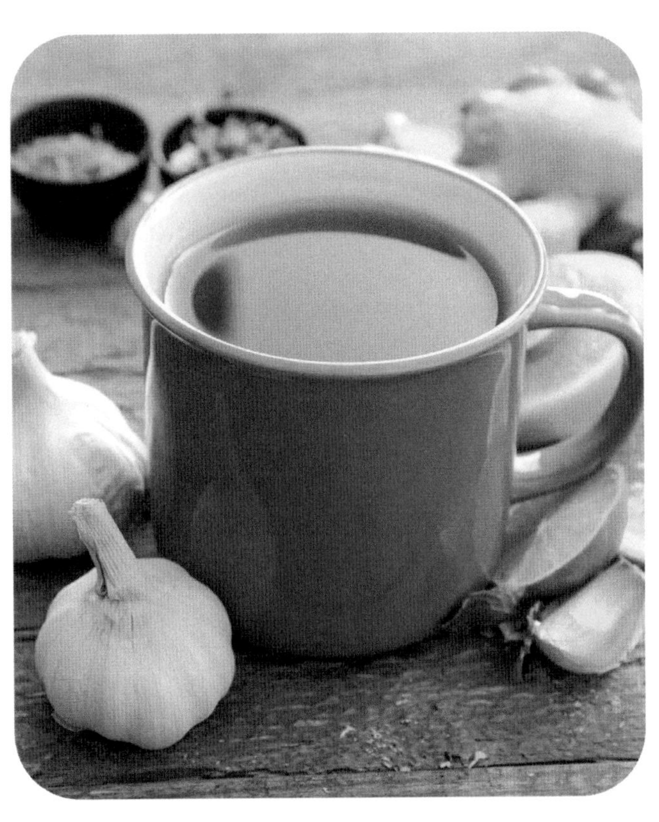

To Prepare:

Put 3 cloves fresh, raw garlic—freshly peeled and crushed—into quart jar.

Fill jar with boiling water and cover immediately (you don't want the steam to escape).

Let cool enough to drink one third. (Add lemon if desired.)

Later in the day drink another third—hot or cold to taste.

Before bed drink the last third, and possibly even eat the pieces of garlic.

Do this for 3 consecutive days.

NOTE: Garlic has many beneficial constituents, chief among them is Allicin. Allicin is anti-viral, antibiotic, anti-fungal, and anti-parasite. It is the only known natural constituent that kills MRSA on contact. It does not suppress your symptoms but will systemically address the cause of them.

Pine Needle Tea & Syrup

Pine packs a hefty punch of immune-boosting properties as a superior source of vitamin C, vitamin A, antioxidants, and it is anti-inflammatory. Folk medicine swears by this as a reliever of chest congestion and sore throats. Pine is an expectorant, meaning it helps to loosen mucus so that it can be coughed up and released. It is a circulatory stimulant, has antimicrobial properties, and is a mild diuretic so it will help flush your kidneys. Pregnant women should not drink pine tea.

You will need:

- good clean water
- raw local honey
- wild foraged pine needles with pinecone buds

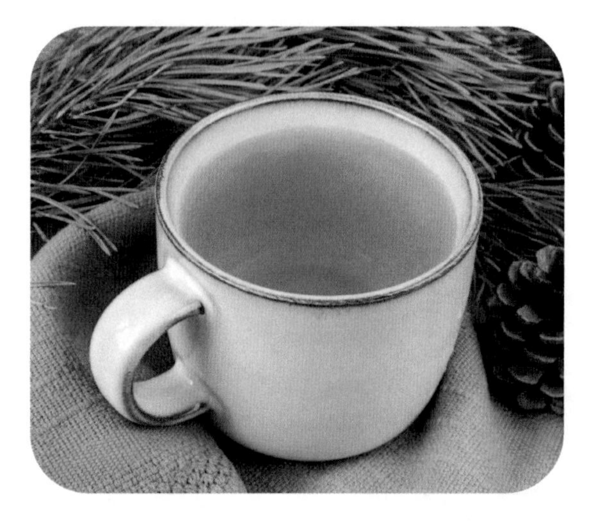

Gather pine branches with needles. Fresh off the tree is best, but I love the after-storm gathering of guilt-free medicine from the forest floor. Inspect and remove any legged creatures and set free outside.

After you inspect the fronds, brush your arm, skin, and face (any exposed skin) with the side of the needles in a slow and comforting way. This stimulates your vagus nerve and immediately calms the nervous system and can induce better sleep, digestion, states of being, and even cause euphoria. If you feel like it, give thanks for the medicine you are about to prepare.

Fill a stock pot with at least ½ gallon water and lightly simmer pine needles in the uncovered pot for an hour or so. You will be able to tell how strong it will taste by how dark the tea becomes. Experiment with brew strength. It's not going to benefit you if you brew it too strong and end up pouring it out. Start small and short and build from there. The longer the simmer, the more benefits in your tea. When done simmering, strain out the pine material, leaving only the tea.

At this point you can leave it as tea and keep jarred in fridge for a month or more. It's great hot or cold. Or, you can add ¼ water volume in local, raw honey and simmer down to thicken to a syrup over very low heat. Take this syrup as needed with a dropper or add to your favorite tea as a sweetener. Refrigerate up to one month.

Zucchini Almond Cake

(Adapted from *The Gluten-Free Almond Flour Cookbook* by Elana Amsterdam.)

This is one cake I bake ahead to take on long car rides and camping. It is basically guilt free. You will never ever miss gluten chocolate cake again, I promise.

Ingredients:

- 2 C almond flour
- ½ t sea salt
- ½ t baking soda
- 1 T cinnamon
- ½ t chipotle pepper, ground
- ½ t chai spice
- 2 T raw cacao
- ¼ C olive oil
- ½ C raw agave (I use dark)
- 2 eggs
- 1 C grated zucchini (or 2-3 overripe bananas)
- ½ C pecans or walnuts, chopped

To Prepare:

Preheat oven to 350°F.

Coat springform pan with coconut oil.

Combine all ingredients together and pour into pan.

Bake about 1 hour, checking for doneness with a toothpick in the center.

Release pan's spring side and cool.

Serve with fruit on top, or whipped cream, or nothing at all.

Stores well on the counter for a day or two but will retain its heavenly, moist texture better if you cover and refrigerate it.

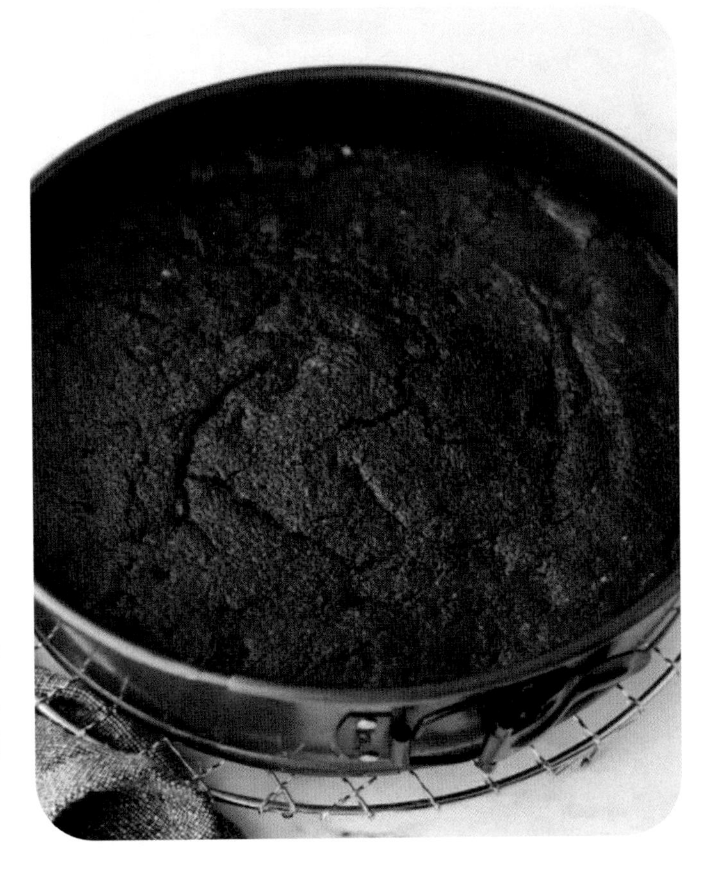

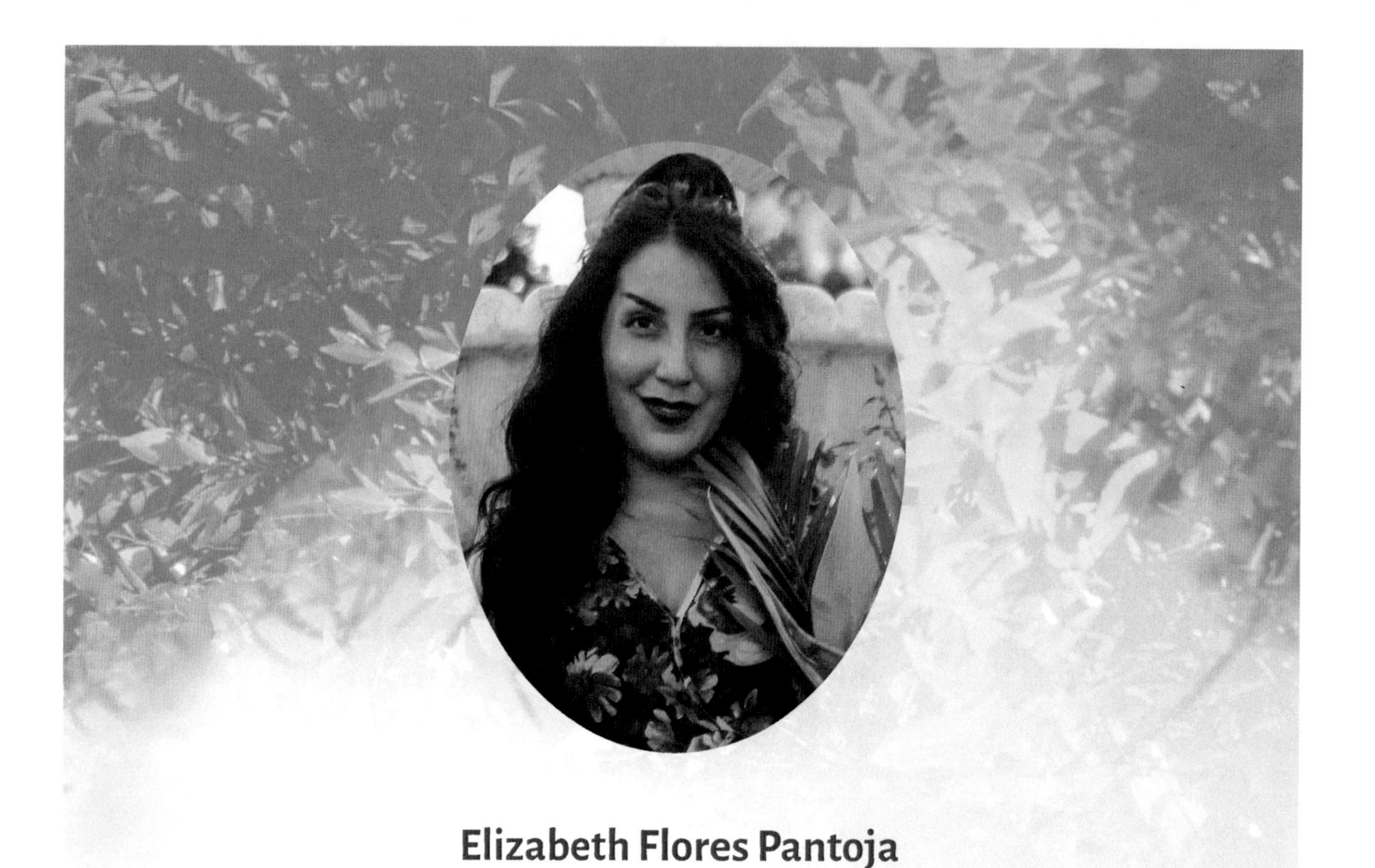

Elizabeth Flores Pantoja

My love for art goes as far back as I can remember. My childhood dreams of being an artist would come to halt when I gave birth to my daughter at the age of16. Through life's challenges, I graduated high school and later received my bachelor's degree in Business.

After college, while transitioning into a healthier lifestyle, I discovered a creative way of intertwining food and art. Flor Bloom, edible arrangements allowed me to reunite with my long-lost love for art.

Embracing my gifts and honoring my natural talents has been a life-long journey. I am an artist, I have always been an artist, and I choose to flourish creatively, with purpose in a way that honors my body, myself, my daughter and everything that mother earth gives us. Food art has allowed me to live life in full bloom, one beautiful floral arrangement at a time.

Email: Inflorbloom@yahoo.com
Instagram: Flor_Bloom
Tiktok: Flor.bloom
Facebook: Flor Bloom

18

Living Life in Flor Bloom

Elizabeth Flores Pantoja

"Living life in full bloom, one Flor arrangement at a time!"

~ Elizabeth Flores Pantoja

Flor bloom bloomed into existence when I finally embraced my passion for food art. As a young girl, I enjoyed sketching, painting roses and sculpting flowers out of clay. When asked what I would be when I grew up, I would always say "an artist." Who would have known that my childhood dreams of being an artist would come to halt when I made choices that would lead my life in a different direction?

At the young age of 16, while still in high school I became a mother and a wife. My free time involved taking care of my baby Lorely, my husband, cooking, cleaning, and homework. I wish I could say that my story was all flowers and butterflies, but I survived an abusive relationship and was divorced shortly after high school. As a single mother, life would continue to challenge me in many ways, but I now had a reason to keep striving stronger than ever, my daughter.

After high school, I considered going to school for art or culinary. Art was a given and was clearly my first choice. My second choice was culinary. Being the oldest of five, I spent a lot of time in the kitchen helping my mother cook, authentically delicious, Mexican meals for the family. I was also a huge fan of the Food Network channel and loved watching Cake Wars. Naturally, culinary felt like the next best career choice.

Unfortunately, neither of my top choices would be pursued; I was heavily influenced by my friends and family to go to school for something that would, "pay well," a "real job" because I needed to pursue a "real career." So, my college journey began, and after having changed my major twice; I graduated with my bachelor's degree in Business Administration.

Over a decade later, fresh out of college, my heart still yearned with the idea that my passion for art was not completely over. To my surprise, art found its way back into my life in a very transitional point in my health journey but this time in a different form. After college, my free time drastically increased, and I spent hours, days, binge-watching food and health documentaries. After doing some research and planning, I set new health goals and started implementing small changes. My daughter and I began to adjust our diet to incorporate healthier, wholesome, nutritional ingredients with every meal. As I transitioned into this new lifestyle, I discovered a creative way of intertwining food and art.

Fortunately, thanks to my mother, I knew how to cook but my new challenge was to recreate mama's recipes but healthier. As a result, I began to experiment in the kitchen, and felt a major responsibility to make some healthy adjustments. The big question was, how was I going to make traditional Mexican meals meat-free, vegetarian or plant-based? Not to mention, adjusting generational, passed-down recipes is a huge no-no and goes against very traditional Mexican cuisine and culture.

Regardless of the lack of support from family and friends, I stuck to the plan and was determined to create meals that even my family would come to love. I started by incorporating more mushrooms and legumes into our diet. I also experimented with different colorful, seasonal, fruits and vegetables from local farmer's markets. Like flowers in full bloom, my creativity sprung back stronger than ever! I began by making roses out of avocados, hand-crafted flowers out of mangos, jicamas, carrots, persimmons and other produce. Every dish had my signature edible rose and I became obsessed with the way food art enhanced my dishes, giving them vibrance, beauty and life.

Ultimately, health can be challenging but it doesn't have to be. Loving our bodies through food should come easy! Over the years, my daughter and I have learned that making healthier choices comes easiest when we allow ourselves to get creative, pick our own ingredients and make our own meals with love. Cooking is an art form and creating homecooked meals allows you to really see what you're feeding your temple. It's truly amazing how food presentation can make the biggest difference in the way healthy food is portrayed. We eat first with our eyes, which explains why it's easier to adjust and transition into eating healthier through food art. My vision is simple; healthy, and nourishing foods don't have to be intimidating; on the contrary, they should be inviting, beautiful and delicioso!

Furthermore, creating food art is therapeutic, playing with different colors, textures and flavors is meditative. It allows you to fully immerse and tap into all your senses. In the floral, food creation process, your heartbeat slows, and your hands play, twist and fold ever so delicately. In many ways, food art reminds me of my younger self, that little artist. I sketch/draw my vision for an arrangement, pick the produce, choose the colors, flavors and textures, and create floral arrangements that allow me step back into those special moments of being young, and making roses out of clay.

Fast forward to now, what started in the kitchen while experimenting with healthy, creative savory, Mexican meals, turned into a deep, sweet, passion for Mexican-inspired, edible arrangements. Flor Bloom, Artisan Edible arrangements bloomed into existence the Summer of 2022. As a Latina, women-owned, mother-daughter, small business we specialize in creating elegant, luxurious, vibrant, delicious customized, hand-crafted, and hand-carved edible arrangements (including vegan & vegetarian options), for those special occasions. We offer fruit baskets, fruit boards, fruit cakes, fruit platters and cater large fruit boards & fruit tables arrangements.

Connecting the dots backwards, Flor bloom bloomed out of the moments I spent in the kitchen, creating meals with my mother, the years spent working in restaurants, the chefs that inspired me and the people that empowered me to become the artist I am today.

Finally, I have come to understand that what is yours will always find its way back to you and that some things aren't taught, you are just born with these God-given-talents. Embracing and honoring my natural gifts and authentic skills has been a life-long journey. I'm now at a point in my life where I choose to embrace my gifts wholeheartedly. My values are now in alignment with my life's-work. It's taken me years to realize something I've always known.. I am an artist! I have always been an artist, and I choose to flourish creatively, with purpose in a way that honors my body, myself, my daughter and everything that mother earth gives us.

I choose to live my life in full bloom one beautiful floral arrangement at a time.

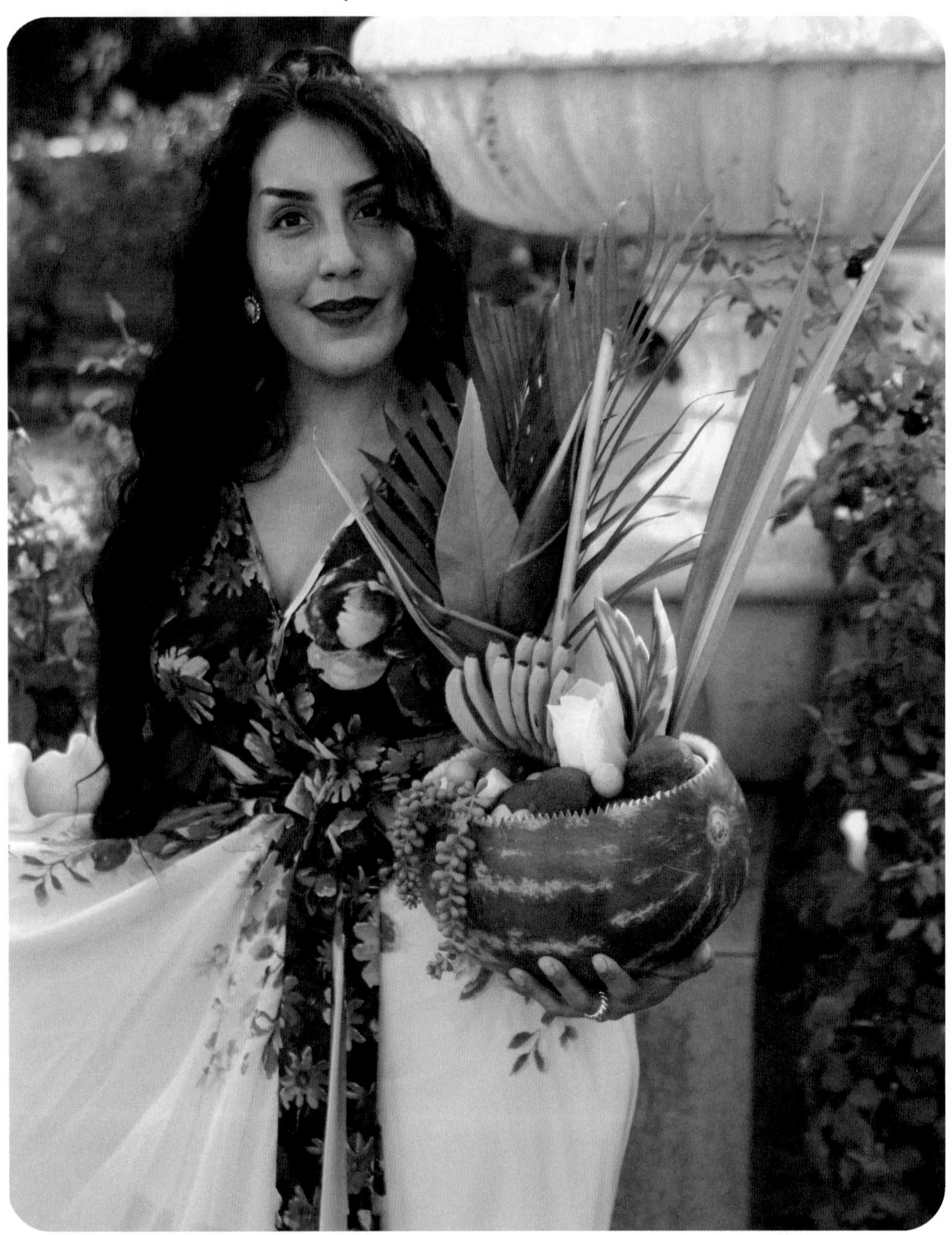

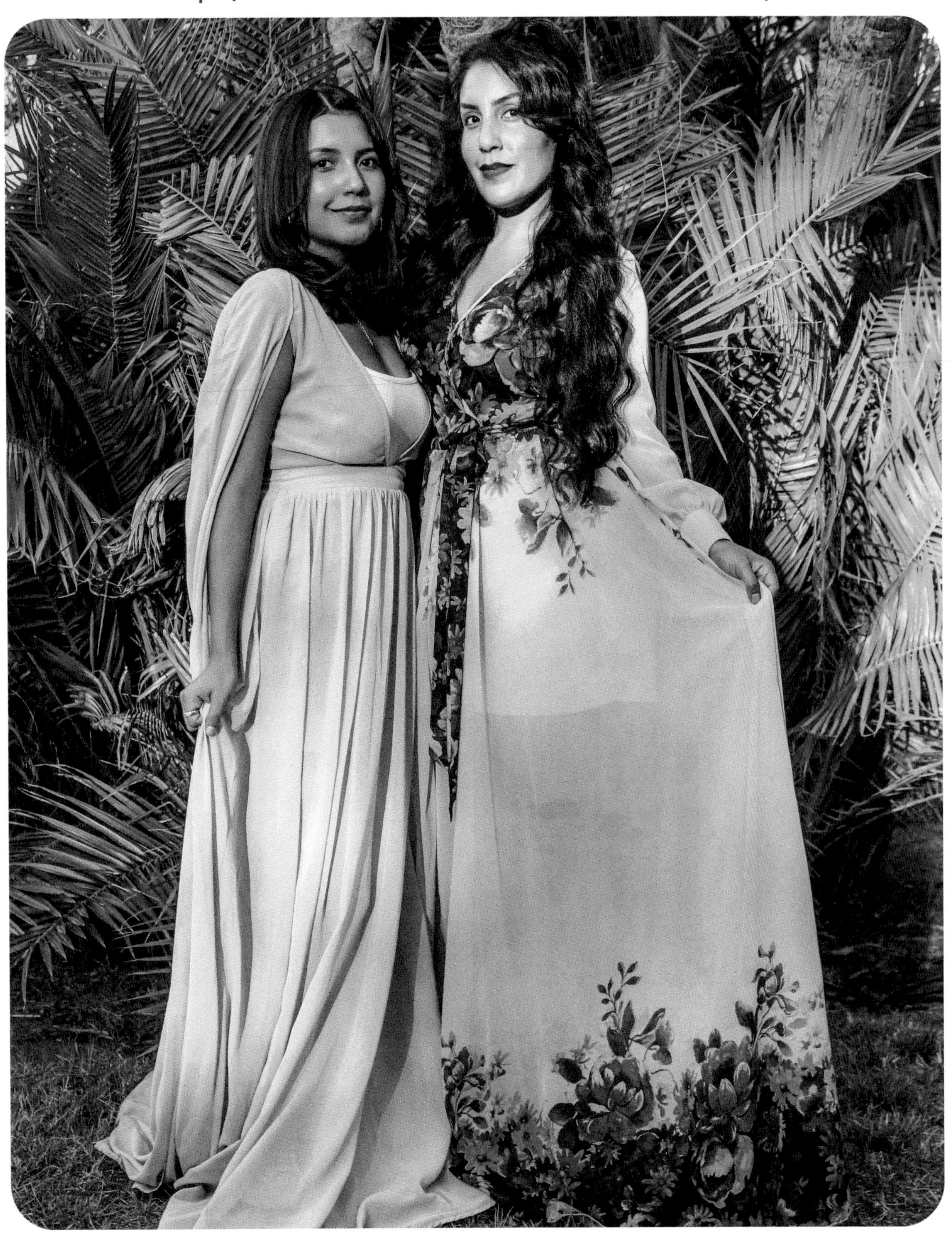

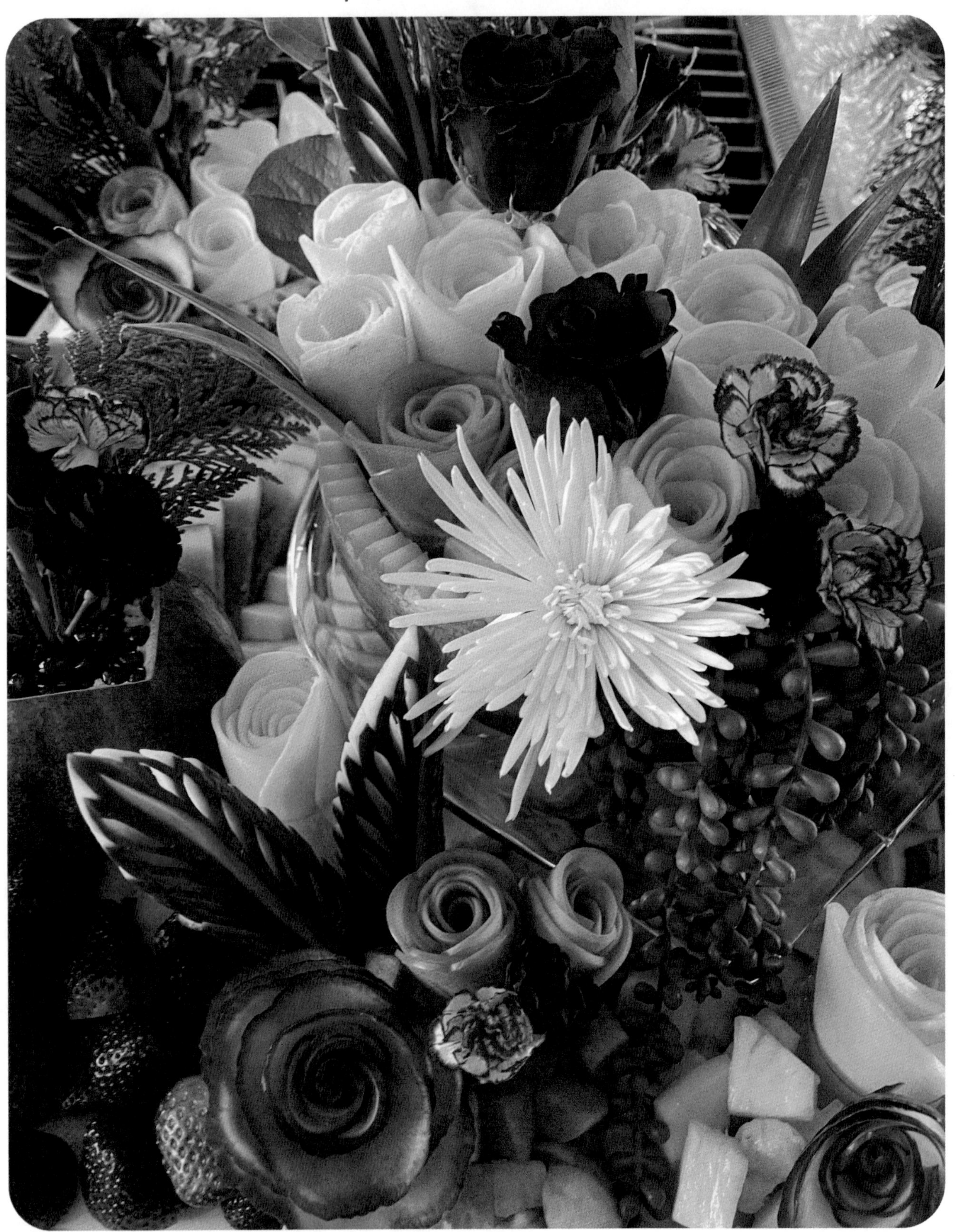

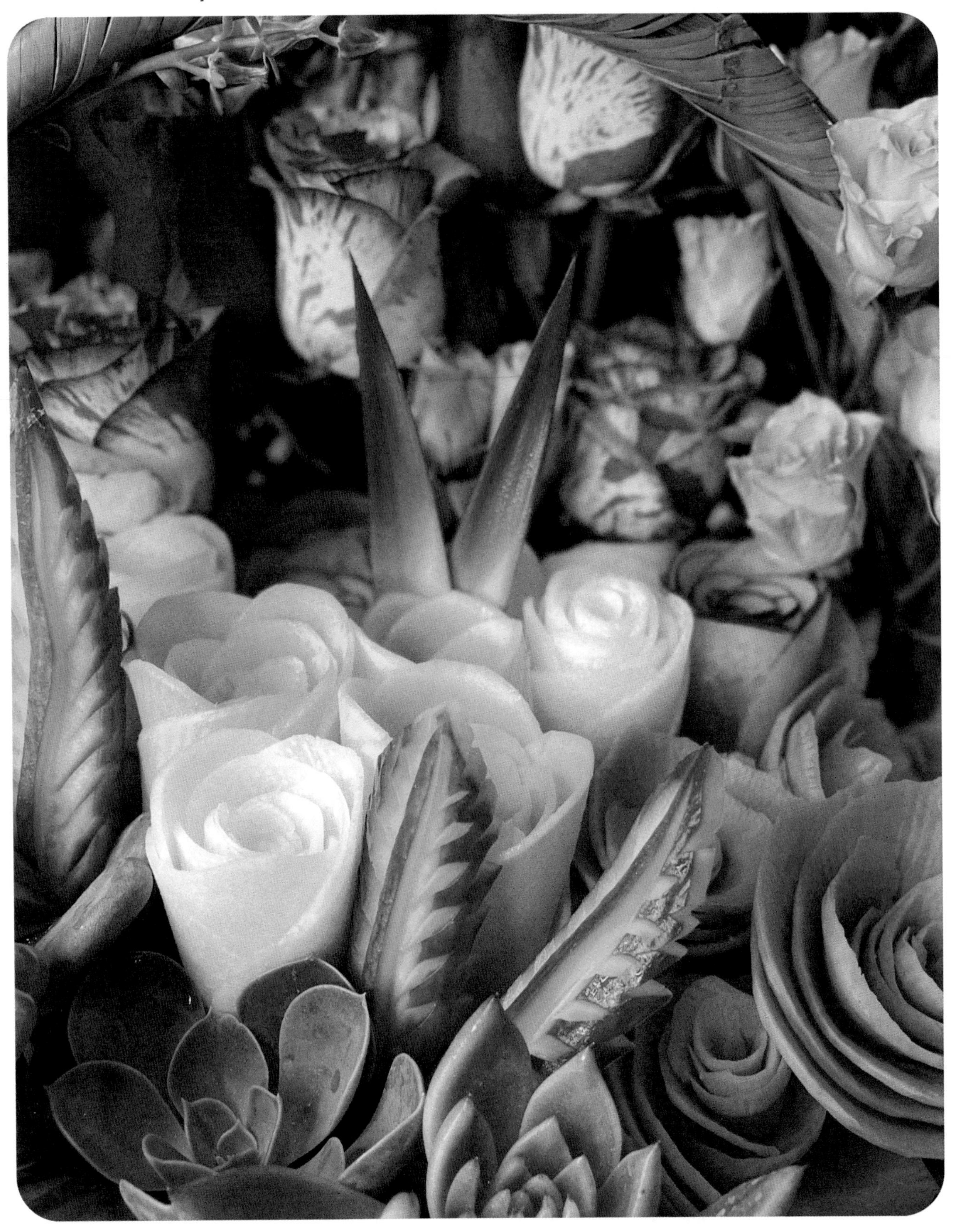

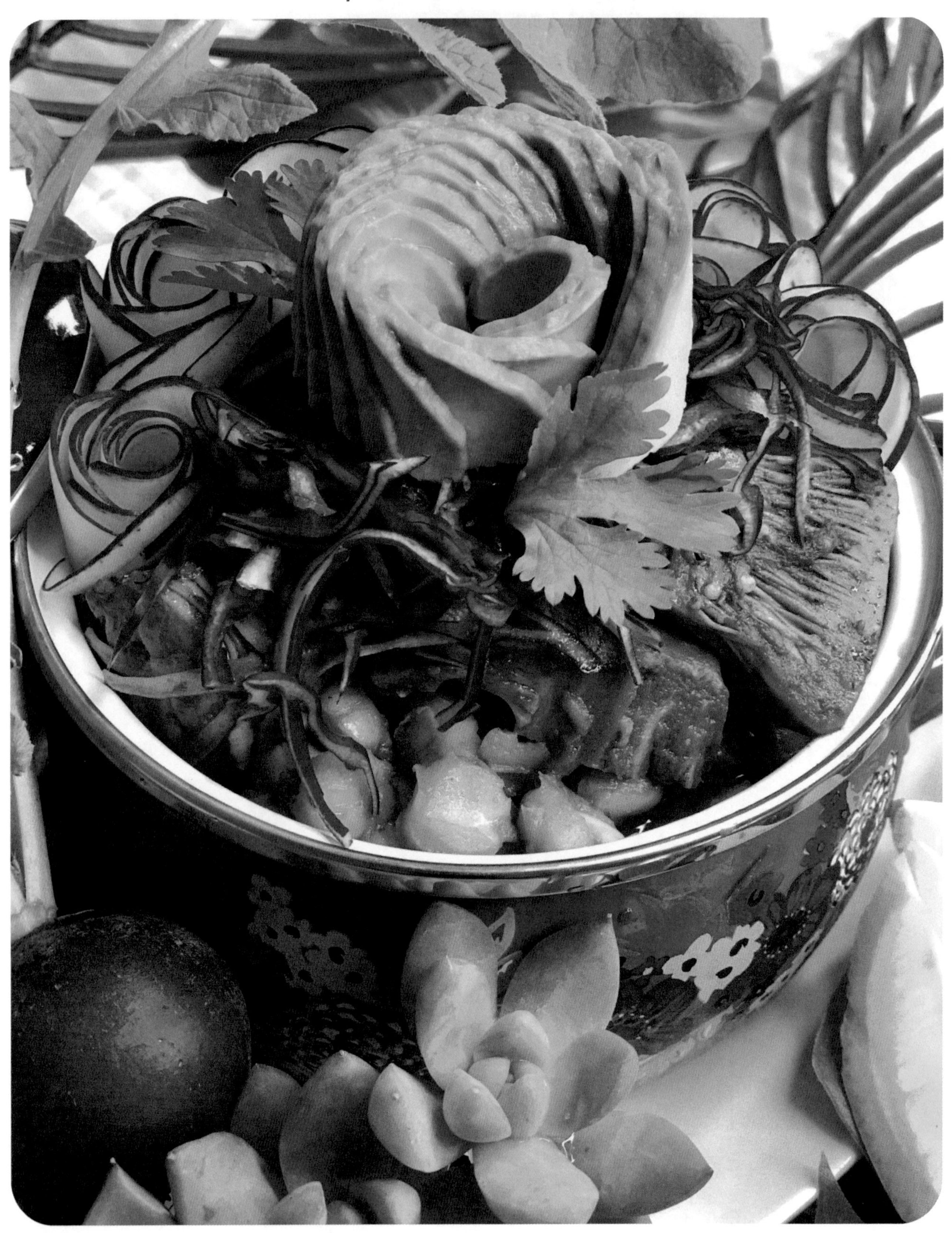

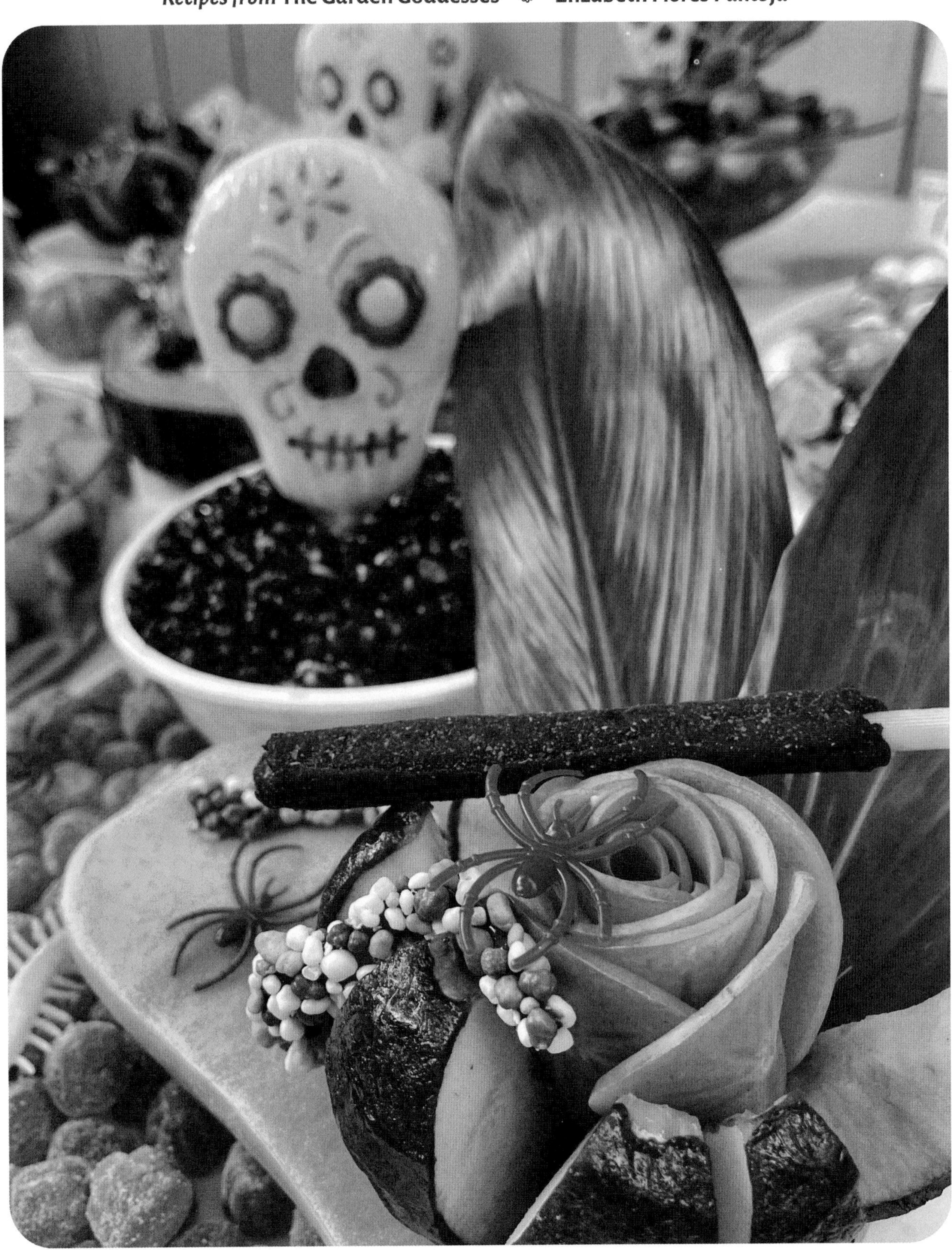

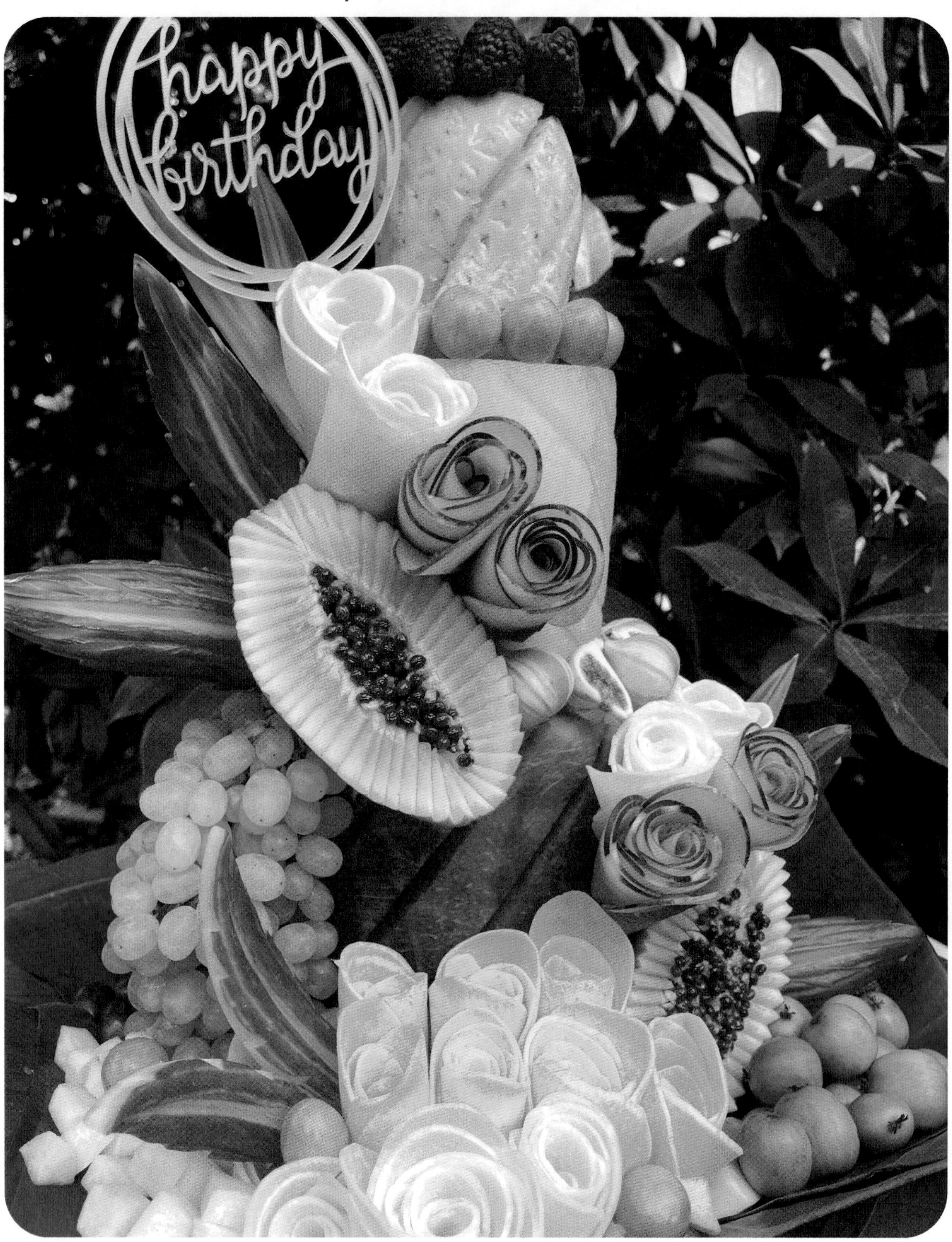
happy
birthday

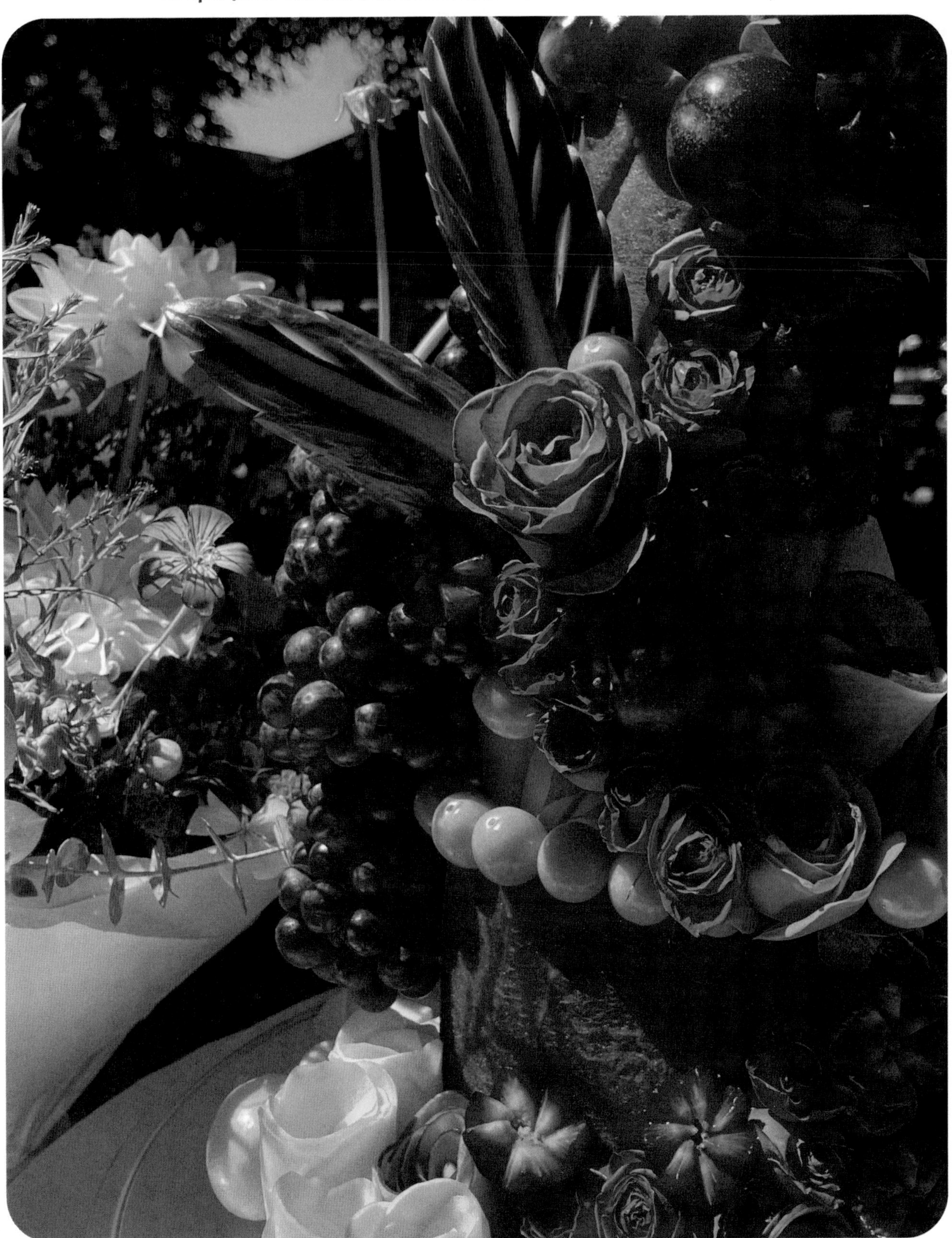

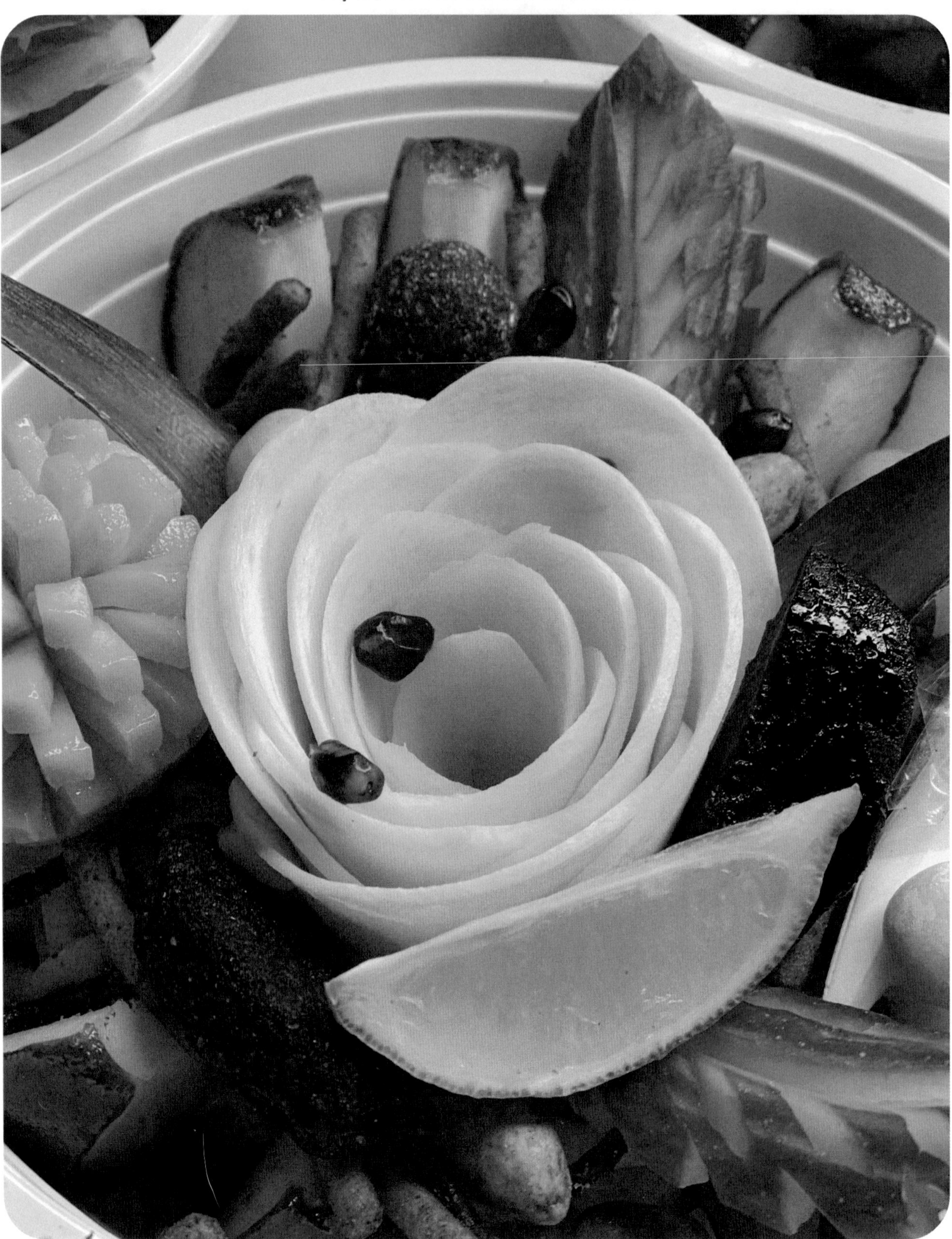

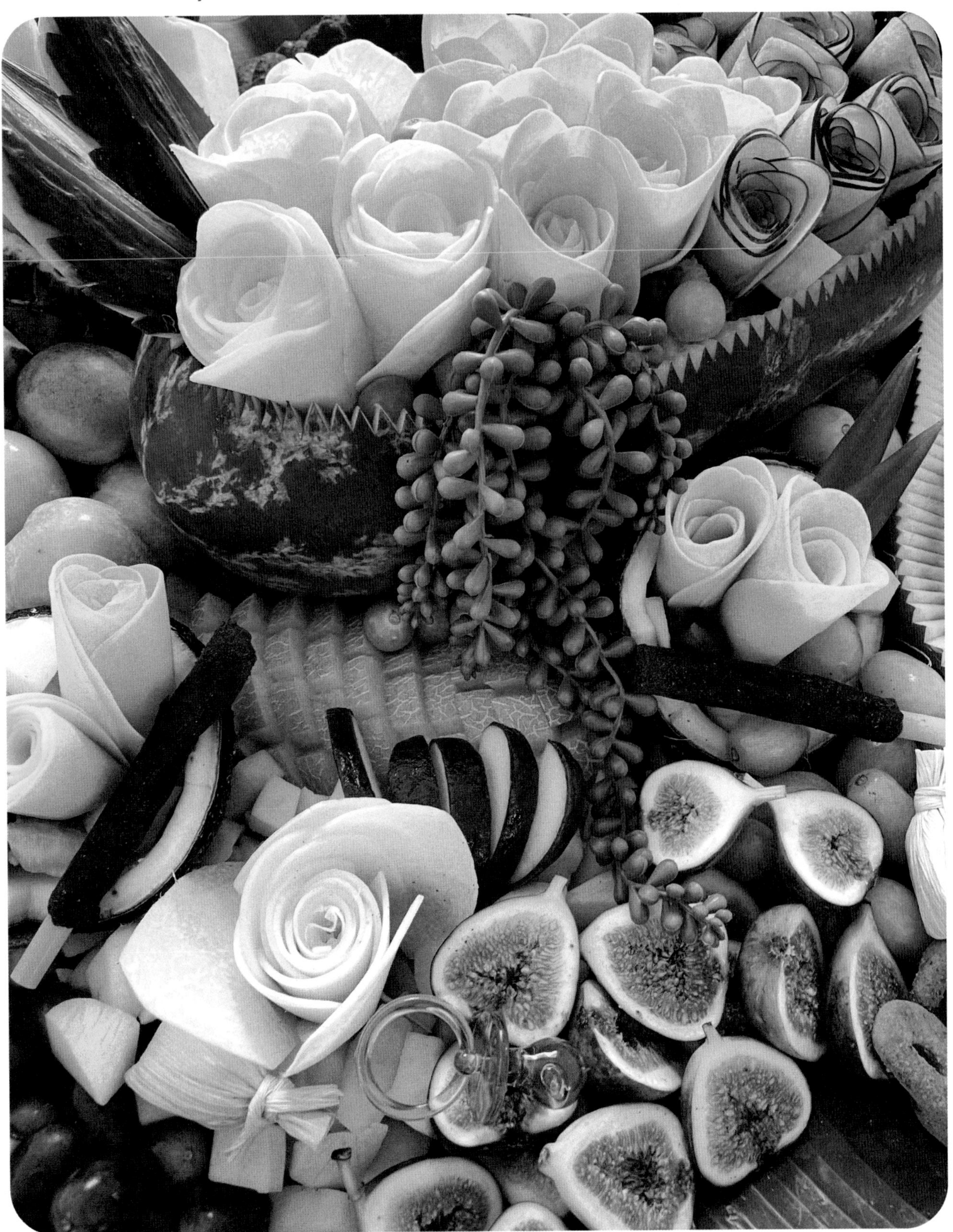

We're honoring each season
and appreciating the bounty
of each harvest.

~ The Society of the Garden Goddesses®

Painting by Masha Lewis

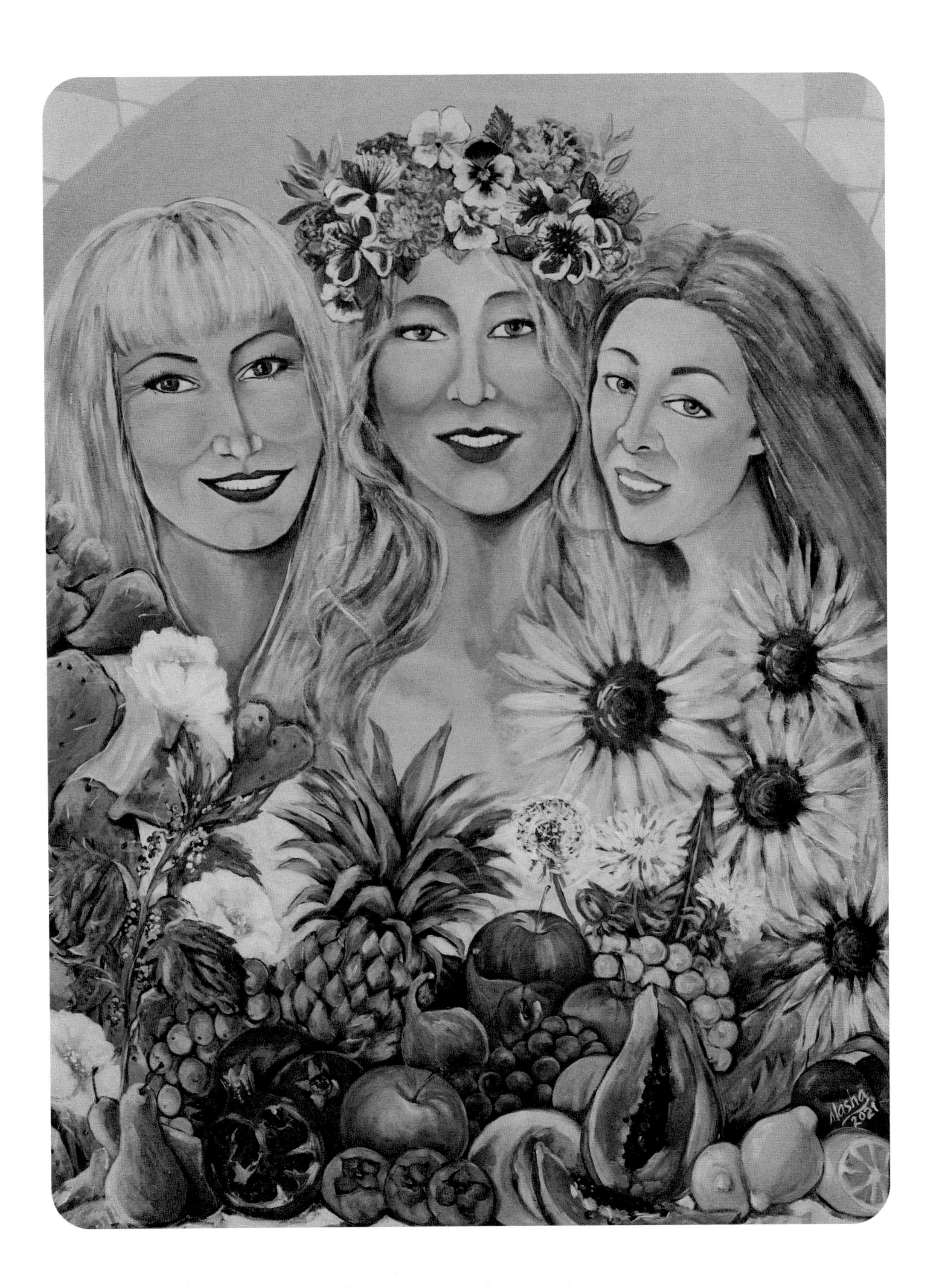
Masha
2021

Made in the USA
Coppell, TX
04 November 2023